BEYOND WOR.

Literature and
Medicine Series

STATEMENT OF PURPOSE: The art of writing and the science
of medicine offer very different approaches to some of the
most intense and mysterious human experiences. The Literature and Medicine series, jointly sponsored by the University
of New Mexico Press and the University of New Mexico's
Health Sciences Center, brings together these two ways of
understanding. Comprising fiction and creative nonfiction,
the series showcases stories that explore the nature of health
and healing and the texture of the experience of illness.

ADVISORY EDITORS: Elizabeth Hadas, Frank Huyler, M.D.,
and David P. Sklar, M.D.

Beyond Words

———

ILLNESS AND THE LIMITS OF EXPRESSION

———

KATHLYN CONWAY

———

University of New Mexico Press
Albuquerque

University of New Mexico Press edition published 2013

by arrangement with the author.

Printed in the United States of America

18 17 16 15 14 13   1 2 3 4 5 6

Library of Congress Cataloging-in-Publication Data

Conway, Kathlyn.
Beyond words : illness and the limits of expression / Kathlyn Conway.
p. cm. — (Literature and medicine series)
Originally published as: Illness and the limits of expression. Ann Arbor : University
of Michigan Press, c2007.
Includes bibliographical references and index.
Summary: "Author Kathlyn Conway, a three-time cancer survivor, believes that
the triumphalist approach to writing about illness fails to do justice to the shattering
experience of disease. By wrestling with the challenge of writing about the reality of
serious illness and injury, she argues, writers can offer a truer picture of the complex
relationship between body and mind"—Provided by publisher.
ISBN 978-0-8263-5324-5 (pbk. : alk. paper) — ISBN 978-0-8263-5325-2 (electronic)
I. Conway, Kathlyn. Illness and the limits of expression. II. Title.
III. Series: Literature and medicine series (Albuquerque, N.M.)
[DNLM: 1. Chronic Disease—psychology—Personal Narratives. 2. Attitude
to Health—Personal Narratives. 3. Catastrophic Illness—psychology—Personal
Narratives. 4. Critical Illness—psychology—Personal Narratives. 5. Medicine in
Literature—Personal Narratives. WT 500]

610—dc23   2012048009

TO DAVID, ZACH, AND MOLLY
AND IN MEMORY OF MY SISTER, CHRIS

– Contents –

– Acknowledgments –

The most gratifying part of writing this book has been the chance to work out my ideas in discussion with people whose intelligence and insight I greatly value. My deepest gratitude in this regard is to David Rosner. In his unassuming way he let me know what didn't work about this project and then what did. During our many conversations about this book he invariably encouraged, challenged, and energized me.

Peter Dimock, whose strength as an editor is his ability to get to the heart of a manuscript and grasp its essence, helped me understand what I was trying to say and insisted I not shrink from saying it. Jonathan Cobb is every writer's dream of a close reader. He took a great deal of time he didn't have to consider with me the overall shape of this book and then to read every word carefully, catching my lapses in logic and my infelicitous phrasing, while always remaining supportive. I thank them both for their expertise, generosity, and especially their friendship.

My editors at the University of Michigan Press were equally helpful. Howard Markel quickly and enthusiastically embraced this project as one that offered a new perspective on illness narratives. Alex Stern remained an unfailingly astute reader at every stage of this book's evolution. Raphael Allen worked with me to place the books I discuss in a cultural context. Mary Erwin lent her expert eye and valuable insights to the final stages of this book.

As always in our long friendship Dennis Marnon was generous in his encouragement and keen in his insights. Gina Hens-Piazza lent her expert skills as a reader to this project, adding yet another role to the many she has played in my life for over forty years. Other friends offered invaluable comments and help: Rita Charon, Tom

Engelhardt, Bonnie Gitlin, Laura Kogel, Deborah Luepnitz, Joan Milano, and Jim O'Brien. Many more discussed this project with me and offered their support. I thank them as well.

As with my first book, Zach and Molly cheered me on. This time, as adults, they also offered their own thoughts on the subject of narrative and illness. I thank them for this and for so much more.

– Foreword –

Alexandra Minna Stern
Howard Markel

At a time when the memoir rivals, and some would argue has replaced, the novel as America's favorite literary genre, Kathy Conway offers a critical evaluation of autobiographical illness narratives. A psychotherapist attuned to the poignancy and problems of human communication who herself has experienced cancer diagnosis and treatment three times, Conway is uniquely poised to employ a mix of analytical, literary, and psychoanalytic skills to challenge the all-pervasive "triumph narrative" of illness.

Yet Conway's anatomy of the illness memoir is far from a denigration or caricature of the genre. Rather it is a subtle and probing exploration of the compulsion to tell stories of triumph, closure, and redemption, even by those with conditions likely to kill or permanently incapacitate them, and of the limits of language to express physical and psychological pain. Conway asks why the impulse to plot illness stories as tales of self-realization or personal transcendence is so overwhelming in today's society. Conway notes that even when she wrote her first book, *Ordinary Life: A Memoir of Illness* as a conscious counternarrative to conventional forms, she felt the inexorable pull of the triumph myth.

In this erudite literary study, Conway questions the idea that suffering through chemotherapy, facing a chronic disease, or negotiating day-to-day life with a disability necessarily makes one a better person. In elegantly written and succinct prose, Conway interweaves a critique that connects the cultural weight of the Christian story of rebirth, the Horatio Alger myth of self-improvement, and a New Age belief that spiritual awareness results in superior health, to American society's fear and denial of dying and death.

Conway navigates the reader through a wide range of memoirs, diaries, and autobiographical writings in order to closely examine how writers understand themselves as subjects of illness and disability. In so doing, she lays bare the landscape of illness narratives. Conway explores how putting words to paper can empower those who are ill, even as language can betray the most creative writers. Indeed, sometimes language—whether analogy, metaphor, or other literary device—simply fails to describe or evoke an individual's authentic experience of physical or psychological suffering. As she points out, the silence that results can itself be a meaningful (although often ignored) response to the poverty of linguistic expression.

Conway's honest and unflinching rejection on the "lost totality" or "catastrophe" experienced by persons with a disease or a disabling condition is refreshing, unsettling, and deeply moving. With its sophisticated focus on a particular literary genre *Beyond Words* nonetheless raises universal questions about expression and what it means to be human.

BEYOND WORDS

Introduction

My interest in illness narratives began in 1993 while I was receiving chemotherapy for breast cancer. Feeling devastated by the experience and unhelped by the many stories offered me as inspiration—the eighty-year-old woman who looked gorgeous after three cancers, the thirty-five-year-old who jogged five miles a day during chemo—I searched for stories written by people like me whose emotional resources were strained to the limit and who were trying with everything they had just to cope. I felt that if there were writers who spoke plainly about what serious illness is really like, then I could learn something from them about how to endure suffering.

I found a plethora of books about illness and disability in which their authors attempt to describe and make sense of a range of devastating bodily experiences. Yet most of these books left me unsatisfied. They fall into the category of what are described as narratives of triumph. In them, the author, after the initial shock and devastation of receiving a serious diagnosis or suffering an accident, and sometimes after a false start or two, finds a comfortable way to cope, and eventually is restored to health or achieves some kind of emotional resolution. These narratives are predictable in plot and moral. The writers of the triumph narrative tend to reflect on their experience relatively little as they go along, reserving reflection for the end. From a position of authority outside the actual experience, they look back and offer this conclusion: if one battles hard and maintains a positive attitude, everything will work out. They often express gratitude for illness as an opportunity for personal growth and offer their advice to the reader: live every day as fully as possible.

These books, while often of interest because of the dramatic nature of their story and the soothing nature of their message, ultimately disappoint. By offering platitudes, they leave the reader with little insight into some of life's most challenging experiences. They decline to struggle over the many questions for which there seem to be few answers. In essence they shrink from the complexity of their experience and focus on one slice of it—the final resolution—which they portray as a triumph that results from determination and a positive attitude. By adhering to the culturally preferred narrative of triumph, authors typically downplay or deny other dimensions of their own experience, particularly the more painful and unmanageable ones. Without a greater acknowledgment of these difficult aspects of illness and disability their triumph seems superficial.

I and many who are ill and disabled have longed for a story that takes us into the darker and less familiar corners of the territory of illness, what Reynolds Price calls "the far side of catastrophe, the dim other side of that high wall that effectively shuts disaster off from the unfazed world."[1] It is a world unto itself, and we who find ourselves there discover that the usual resources for coping are sorely tried. We long to hear from someone who speaks from within personal experience and describes what it is really like to have cancer, to lose a leg, to become blind, or to feel the mind spinning out of control. We long to hear from someone who admits that even enormous love from others does not erase the essential loneliness of illness. We want to hear not clichés but an acknowledgment that illness is not simply an opportunity for personal growth but a soul-wrenching encounter with loss, limitation, and the reality of death. We want to hear from someone who does not go gently into that dark night.

I wrote and published my own memoir[2] in an attempt to describe my experience on the far side of breast cancer. Later, I did discover a group of books—few of them to be found on the shelves of my local bookstore—whose authors had attempted to describe serious illness or injury and explored more fully those questions about life that resist easy answers. These writers, by reflecting throughout their narratives on the ways illness or accident shattered their selves and altered their lives, push the boundaries of what we can understand about these devastating experiences. Through the lens of their individual struggles they tell us something new. Their accomplishment—itself a kind of triumph—lies not in defeating illness but in a willingness to embrace all aspects of the experience and to remain true to themselves throughout.

Interestingly, many of the authors of these books begin with a statement of how few good books about illness they have found. Reynolds Price reports that he found only a "very slim row of sane printed matter which comes from the far side of catastrophe."[3] While these protestations may be, as Nancy Mairs[4] suggests, a way authors advertise their own books, they still reflect a genuine frustration with how little attention is paid to the more challenging and difficult aspects of the experience.

These narratives, I believe, have important cultural significance. In describing, without needing to resolve, their conflicts between battling and giving up, between finding meaning and not, between denying and acknowledging death, their authors suggest a different cultural conception of serious illness and disability. In contemporary American culture, where a denial of illness and an unwillingness to face death is pervasive, they suggest not just a better technique for managing illness but a place outside of technique where author and reader alike can simply reflect on these very human experiences.

While reading these personal narratives that depict the more difficult aspects of illness and disability, I discovered that their authors not only push the boundaries of what we can understand about illness and disability, but also describe their confrontation with the limits of language and literary form for representing pain, suffering, and awareness of mortality. I will argue, using these texts as evidence, that for those who are ill or disabled, writing frustrates as much as it heals. Even as these writers find language and form for their experience, they discover that something of its emotional intensity slips away in the telling of their story. Still, their attempts are invaluable; they marshal all their resources of intellect, will, and humor to face, and allow us to face, the limits of the self and its expression in language.

Memoirs whose authors struggle to describe in detail the damage to their sense of self and to their life, while still a distinct minority among illness narratives, are receiving a great deal of attention in some circles. Literature about illness is now extensively analyzed and promoted as part of a new patient-centered ethos being advocated in many medical schools. Personal stories about illness are read by those who are ill and their families, hospice and health care workers, the general public, and medical students in humanities programs. In addition, literature about illness has increasingly become the subject of inquiry in academic departments like English literature, anthropology, and medical humanities as well as an object of controversy among literary critics.

Why this boom in interest? Although more and more people survive serious illness and thus face questions about how to live with physical limitations and a greater awareness of mortality, contemporary mainstream American culture provides little help with these questions. The emphasis on youth, physical strength, and beauty not only constitutes a denial of illness and dying but also causes illness to be viewed as anomalous and relegated to the separate world of medicine. That world—characterized by high-tech treatments, specialization, and sometimes professional indifference—often proves inhospitable to a humane and generous embrace of the frightened person who suffers. In addition, those who have been estranged from religious and community rites and routines that once provided consolation during illness and at the time of death may feel unmoored. Some turn to literature for help.

Most of the available literature, however, as I have said, takes the form of what has come to be called the narrative of triumph. I use this term much in the way Arthur Frank uses the term *restitution narrative* to describe stories that follow this plot line: "Yesterday I was healthy, today I'm sick, but tomorrow I'll be healthy again."[5] This, he believes, is the most pervasive narrative in American popular culture, brought to us in television commercials, magazine advertisements, and hospital brochures.[6] G. Thomas Couser refers to it as the "culturally validated narrative of triumph over adversity"[7] in which, at the end, "the narrators are healed, if not cured" and are "better off at the end than at the beginning."[8] As Couser suggests, the resolution may be restored physical health or the achievement of peace of mind. Such stories center on a certain sort of character: the protagonist in a narrative of triumph possesses traits that will insure a triumphant ending: he or she takes action, battles heroically, and maintains an optimistic attitude.

This dominant tradition in illness narratives, that of the narrative of triumph, finds its written expression in both self-help books and personal memoirs. Straightforward self-help books that deal with the general subject of health often offer stories to prove that the behavior or attitudes they advocate will result in healing. Popular examples include Norman Cousins's *Anatomy of an Illness as Perceived by the Patient*, Bernie Siegel's *Love, Medicine and Miracles*, Andrew Weil's *Spontaneous Healing*, and Deepak Chopra's *Creating Health*.[9] Although some of these books contain useful information, their authors at times betray exaggerated confidence in the prescriptions they offer for warding off death. Chopra, for example, in the course of maintaining that an individual's attitude and emotional state determine his or her health, tells the story of a forty-two-year-old business executive who drops dead of a heart attack while in Chopra's office, not because his arteries are clogged but because of a "spasm of the coronary vessels, directly induced by hostility, resentment, impatience, fear and exaggerated feelings of being indispensable."[10] Chopra reassures another patient, who, after suffering several episodes of ventricular fibrillations fears a lifetime of debt because he has no health insurance, that his bill will be paid. This reduction in anxiety somehow stops his fibrillations; he needs no further treatment and is sent home to live happily ever after.[11]

In *Spontaneous Healing* Andrew Weil relates stories of people who recovered even though their doctors had given up hope. In another age these stories might have been designated miracles; for Weil they are proof that proper behavior and attitude can cure disease. He tells the story of Kristin, who, after two failed bone marrow transplants for aplastic anemia, is expected to die. Refusing to give up, she tries every available treatment and is healthy today, twenty years later. Weil remarks on her "unwavering confidence through her ordeal" and asks rhetorically, "What reserves of healing power did Kristin draw on to reactivate her bone marrow, neutralize whatever was the original cause of the disease, and undo the toxic effects of invasive treatment?"[12]

If sales figures are a good measure, many people read these books and, presumably, derive hope from the notion that they can control their health. When I read such books, however, I feel annoyed. To suggest, for example, that a proper attitude could have prevented or even cured the serious cancers for which I and millions of others have endured surgery, radiation, and chemotherapy denies the gravity of life-threatening illness.

The scientifically dubious and hubristic idea that the right attitude brings a cure holds enormous sway in contemporary American thinking about illness, perhaps because it fits so well with the American belief that anything is possible. In fact, there has been strikingly little questioning of the validity of the notion that positive thinking cures. There have been scientific experiments that have demonstrated the relationship between emotions and health, as indicated by Esther Sternberg in *The Balance Within*.[13] Sternberg reviews experiments demonstrating the physical mechanisms used by the brain and immune system to communicate with each other. However, the notion that positive thinking actually contributes to cure has yet to be substantiated.[14]

Although some psychotherapies encourage people to substitute positive feelings for negative, most psychological theories suggest that ignoring negative feelings is detrimental, that mental health rests upon a person's ability to experience and tolerate the full range of emotions, including—and perhaps especially—difficult, painful, and negative feelings. Sigmund Freud, Carl Jung, Jacques Lacan, and the object relations theorists, for example, all point to the need to face the darker side of life. Nonetheless, the ill continue to be told to think positive thoughts or visualize themselves on a beach, as if banishing painful realities from one's thought is always possible or a sufficient way to deal with an experience as relentlessly demanding of attention as illness.

In *Seeing the Crab* Christina Middlebrook, herself a Jungian analyst, argues that acknowledging the dark side of life actually diminishes fear.[15] She relates the story of a colleague who, consulted because the children in a nursery school were having nightmares, discovered that the teachers and parents "were editing out the evil characters and frightening endings from the fairy tales and nursery rhymes that they read aloud" to the children.[16] When the adults refrained from editing, the children's nightmares stopped. Many of the writers I will discuss reject the triumph narrative precisely because it edits out the dark characters and emotions that they maintain are inevitably part of the story.

In addition to explicit self-help narratives, a vast array of first-person illness narratives are structured as stories of triumph and offer the same message: positive thinking and proper behavior will result in triumph. Sometimes their titles, with their insistence on hope and their denial of negative feelings, render their triumphalist message transparent. Hamilton Jordan, the chief of staff under Jimmy Carter, entitles his book about his three cancers *No Such Thing as a Bad Day*. Vickie Girard writes a book entitled *There's No Place Like Hope*. While the actual story in a triumph narrative may include much that is painful, the conclusion of most narrators, generally offered at the end, is that illness is an opportunity for growth or transformation for which the author is grateful and that life is better than before the illness or accident. As Heather Jose, who at twenty-six was diagnosed with first-stage breast cancer, puts it, "This is not what I envisioned for my life, but in many ways it is better."[17]

Most first-person narratives, however, even when essentially triumph stories, tend to be more complex than the stories told to advance a self-help program. John Gunther's classic 1949 book *Death Be Not Proud*, while essentially a triumph story about Gunther's seventeen-year-old son who died from a brain tumor, still describes the roller-coaster experience of recoveries, setbacks, and terror aroused by the slightest worried tone in a doctor's voice.[18] Similarly, Betty Rollins, in her 1976 book *First You Cry*, tells her story as one of triumph, hoping to remove the stigma attached to breast cancer, but she is honest about the anxiety, fear, and losses involved.[19]

Lance Armstrong's more recent *It's Not About the Bike* (co-authored with Sally Jenkins in 2000) looks like the prototypical triumph narrative: Armstrong recovers from advanced testicular cancer to win the Tour de France.[20] But Armstrong manages to acknowledge the darker side of the experience even while adhering to the overall structure of the triumph narrative. He describes what it is like to receive a terrible diagnosis, then to hear bad news become worse news, and finally to undergo a punishing chemotherapy regimen. He does not deny his anger when his sponsor cancels his contract because he assumes Armstrong will not recover, nor does he gloss over the depression he suffered after his treatment ended.

A second and less populated tradition of books looks more squarely at the devastating reality of serious illness or disability. The best-known of these are not personal memoirs but books that reflect more generally on the experience of illness and dying. In her 1969 book *On Death and Dying* Elisabeth Kübler-Ross designated five psychological stages of illness: denial and isolation, anger, bargaining, depression, and acceptance.[21] While her schema has been criticized as overly generalized and simplistic, she deserves credit for encouraging people to face their situations and acknowledge the full range of their emotions. Susan Sontag, in her 1978 book *Illness as Metaphor*, examines the way the language used for illness tends to romanticize, sentimentalize, or misrepresent illness in ways that harm the person who is ill. She argues that illness should be seen for what it really is.[22] In a culture where people rarely witness a death, the popularity of Sherwin Nuland's 1993 book *How We Die* represents a further extension of the desire to abandon imagined scenarios and look unflinchingly at the process of dying. Nuland describes the physical process of dying for those with cancer, heart attacks, stroke, AIDS, and Alzheimer's disease.[23]

This tradition also contains many personal narratives in which the authors explicitly reject the triumph narrative and attempt to tell a story that focuses more deeply on what is devastating about the experience of illness. Implicit in this writing is the suggestion that, while illness is now an acceptable topic of discussion, the difficulties of serious illness are often not. These authors go so far as to suggest that our cultural insistence on triumph can result in harm to patients, contributing at times to a refusal on the part of caretakers to hear reports of pain. As a result, real physical problems are overlooked, bad treatment results, and patients are left feeling isolated and even shunned for their failure to triumph.

As an alternative to the triumph narrative, these writers offer accounts that attempt to record their subjective experience of illness—what it is like to suffer serious damage to one's body. Together these narratives create a space in which the most devastating aspects of the experience of serious illness and dying can be articulated, reflected upon, and shared—the loss of control, ruptures in the self, disruptions in the life story, and questions of meaning in the face of personal annihilation. In these narratives the ill and dying can speak honestly in ways that are often not possible within their families and larger society. They open a much needed conversation about the ways in which the desolation of serious illness and disability cannot be managed as the self-help literature would have it. These writers allow us to stand with them as they face the fundamental human predicament—that in the end we die. They invite us to reflect not only on illness but on the basic human condition.

Over the last few decades or so, as personal memoirs of illness and disability have proliferated, they, along with other artistic representations of illness, have become a subject not just of attention, but sometimes of scorn, among literary critics. A pivotal moment in the history of criticism of art that depicts illness occurred in 1994 when the dance critic Arlene Croce published an article entitled "Discussing the Undiscussable" in the *New Yorker*. In it she uses the term *victim art* to describe a dance performance she actually refused to see. Choreographed by Bill T. Jones, who is HIV positive, the piece includes videotapes of terminally ill people talking about their illness. Croce argued, "I can't review someone I feel sorry for or hopeless about."[24] Her article provoked a huge and often outraged response, not only because Croce was criticizing a performance she had never even seen but also because her response was, as Richard Goldstein put it in the *Village Voice*, "a way to cast aspersions on any artist who dares to address oppression without the saving grace of transcendence."[25]

While critics today do not crassly reject artistic works about illness, a contemptuous and dismissive tone still characterizes much contemporary criticism of personal memoirs. Reviews often begin with what has come to seem formulaic dismissal. The reviewer, like a film critic embarrassed about watching reality shows on TV, must distance him- or herself from the genre. For example, in an essay entitled "What Memory Forgets" Patrick Smith writes, "The memoir trend is not just a publishing ruse to get more people to buy books. It's an intellectual fraud, a cultural fraud, a fraud perpetrated by us, in the end, upon ourselves and our past."[26] Despite his dramatic dismissal, Smith goes on to say, "Having committed several big words to print, let me continue with a gaping contradiction—apparent, not real: We have been treated to some very fine memoirs in the past couple of years."[27] This general scorn for memoir is felt even by those who write them, as Laura Miller comments: "Even people working on their own memoirs will quickly follow up the announcement with a disclaimer explaining that while they hate the form—it's self-indulgent, spurious and so *over*—nevertheless, they are, sheepishly, writing a memoir."[28]

Positive reviews of memoirs about illness almost routinely make the point that the book in question is an exception to the rule that such books are self-indulgent and unworthy of attention. Morris Dickstein writes a glowing review of Sherwin Nuland's *Lost in America*, which contains a long account of Nuland's debilitating depression. Rather than explore the possibilities of memoir for describing illness, Dickstein reminds us once again that it is a suspect form of writing. "In recent decades . . . readers also began devouring therapeutic memoirs of abuse, dysfunction and personal anguish. Like guests on daytime talk shows encouraged to parade their wounds, these tale bearers were judged less by what they achieved than by how much they suffered."[29]

While critics have a right to expect certain standards, the fact that personal narratives of illness and disability evoke such strong reactions suggests that there is something more going on than critical distress over a maudlin genre. Critics often argue that because narratives of illness and disability focus so much on the personal, they fail to open out to wider social or historical issues of concern to the public. I would argue, instead, that the best illness memoirs do open out to consider such issues: some offer a cultural critique of American society, its ideal of the perfect body and its notion that all problems can be fixed; others explore the universal question of living life in the face of death. Furthermore, this criticism ignores a fundamental fact about physical suffering: its essential characteristic is that it cuts a person off from the outside world and turns him or her inward. In fact, this very personal and inward retreat and focus on the body often *is* the story. Perhaps the first question we need to ask directly is whether we consider this inward journey a fitting subject of literature. If we do, then what is it we are asking of these narratives?

Of late there are examples of a less dismissive and more appreciative appraisal of writing about illness. The *Paris Review* has reprinted Virginia Woolf's essay "On Being Ill" and it has been read and widely reviewed as an example of a much needed literature about illness.[30] James Fenton responds to Woolf's contention that we have no literature of illness by offering what he considers excellent examples of such writing in the nineteenth century.[31] Julian Barnes has written a laudatory introduction to Alphonse Daudet's *In the Land of Pain*, celebrating it as an excellent example of effective writing about pain and suffering.[32] In his essay "The Body of Imagination," Leonard Kriegel offers an overview of contemporary books about illness and disability, suggesting that "never before have so many written so well about the afflictions of the body."[33] Joan Didion's *The Year of Magical Thinking*, about the sudden death of her husband, the writer John Gregory Dunne, and the serious illness of her daughter, was widely read, reviewed, and chosen for literary prizes when published in 2005.[34]

A small but growing academic literature focuses on both the actual experience of illness and the nature and conventions of illness narratives. A few studies are generally cited as an introduction. In 1988 the anthropologist and physician Arthur Kleinman published *The Illness Narratives: Suffering, Healing and the Human Condition*, in which he states "that it is possible to talk with patients, even those who are most distressed, about the actual experience of illness, and that witnessing and helping to order that experience can be of therapeutic value."[35] He advocates the use of the patient's story as a way to understand the meaning of illness. In 1991 Kathryn Montgomery Hunter, a professor of English who participated in early efforts to introduce humanities into the medical school curriculum, sees pathographies (patient's stories) as a necessary correction to the overemphasis on other kinds of illness narratives in the medical world—the patient's history and chart, written and published case histories, clinical conferences.[36] Anne Hunsaker Hawkins in *Reconstructing Illness: Studies in Pathography* considers how underlying myths like rebirth, battle, and the journey both give form to, and suggest the meaning of, illness stories.[37] In the *The Wounded Storyteller* Arthur W. Frank views contemporary illness narratives as a postmodern phenomenon representing the patient's reclaiming of his or her voice in the medical dialogue. He sees these stories as falling into three broad categories: narratives of restitution, chaos, and quest. In *Recovering Bodies* Thomas Couser defines the different conventions particular to autobiographical accounts of illness by focusing on four different diseases. All of these writers share a recognition of the need for a renewed focus on the patient's story and its individual and collective function. They also agree that the proliferation of illness memoirs is a recent phenomenon.[38]

More recent scholarship analyzes illness memoirs using the paradigms and language of particular frameworks like postmodernism and postcolonialism. While much of this scholarly work deepens and informs our understanding of writing about illness, a reverence has grown up around illness narratives that in itself can block a deeper exploration of their value and limits.

I would like to focus on those illness and disability narratives that depict the complex experience of self. While these narratives are important for what they tell us about an individual's experience, they also represent a collective questioning of the validity of the culturally sanctioned triumph narrative and of the notion that all illness can be managed or transcended. Taken together, they map a more complex story than that of triumph, by paying close attention to the difficult and often unmanageable reality of physical and emotional pain and suffering.

Different historical periods produce different stories. In the Western world, before modern advances in medicine, when little was available in the way of cure, the story of Christianity was often the lens through which illness was viewed. It suggested that people do not control but must accept their fate and that suffering has meaning: it was the path to redemption. With the discovery of antibiotics and the advent of other modern medical treatments the triumph narrative began to gain ground: recovery, even miraculous recovery and a return to health, was sometimes possible. Paradoxically, however, although the cures and treatments of modern medicine allow more people to survive, the narrative of triumph typically fails to capture what survival entails. First of all, treatments like chemotherapy, heart surgery, and organ transplants are themselves debilitating. Second, illness or treatment may be followed by recurrences, secondary illnesses, or disabilities. While successful treatment can be seen as a story of medical triumph, for the individual it is also frequently a matter of continued treatment, further monitoring, susceptibility to further disease, and awareness of contingency. Those who survive know they are not in control, that illness happens, bodies break down. Surviving serious illness may be a triumph of sorts, but living with the reality of physical limitation and a greater awareness of mortality is sobering and challenging.

In an earlier era I would no longer be alive. At twenty-six I was one of the first generation of people successfully treated with radiation for Hodgkin's disease. At forty-three I was treated with chemotherapy for a first-stage breast cancer and then at forty-six with chemo for Hodgkin's disease again. My husband has chronic asthma and was recently diagnosed with myasthenia gravis, an autoimmune neurological disease that in the past would have been debilitating. We and increasing numbers of people now survive illnesses that we might not have survived in the past. Many of us live less with a sense of pride for surviving than with the sense of how completely our lives and psyches have been thrown into turmoil. We see our survival not as the result of our having battled bravely or having adopted the proper attitude, but as our having been lucky enough to be diagnosed with treatable diseases in a country where treatments are available and where we have adequate health insurance. Given the proliferation of experiences like these, we need a different story.

The books I have chosen to discuss in the pages that follow represent the beginnings of that different kind of story. Their authors do not gloss over the devastating experiences and damaged sense of self that grave illness or disability often entails. They question the conventions of the triumph story and, within their stories, they reflect on, wrestle with, or sometimes experiment with language and form in an attempt to accurately represent the essence of their experience. Not surprisingly, many of these books are written by professional writers who became ill or disabled; by definition they are attuned to questions of language and narrative. I do not attempt to cover all illnesses, and in fact I refer over and over again to certain books that focus on the representation of the self that is so critical to understanding the experience of serious illness. Nor do I focus on the distinctions between different illnesses and disabilities. Instead, in an attempt to define a broader and more collective experience of illness, I look to see what of an individual's experience is shared by others.

Although I focus primarily on contemporary books, I also discuss at some length writers such as the nineteenth-century French novelist Alphonse Daudet, who describes his life with syphilis (recently published as *In the Land of Pain*) and the twentieth-century British novelist and essayist Virginia Woolf (particularly her diaries and her 1930 essay, "On Being Ill"), who writes about her experience with manic depression.[39] The issues with which they struggle are uncannily similar to those contemporary illness writers focus on. I also refer to stories of the Holocaust, because in them people struggle to describe an experience that seems beyond description.

I emphasize throughout how devastating is the experience of serious illness or injury, and how they can throw a person's life into chaos and bring home the reality of death. It is important to note, however, that not everyone would frame the experience as devastating in the way I suggest many do. Many people born with a serious disability, for example, would not describe their disability as a tragedy but simply as a part of how life is for them. Others have made sufficient adjustments to their physical disability so that the limits on them appear no more serious than other kinds of limits people encounter in life. These people do not write the kind of story I am describing. So let me be clear. I do not wish to impose a particular narrative on all illness or disability experiences. Nevertheless, I maintain, many who are ill or disabled do find the experience devastating even as they are asked to view it as an occasion for triumph.

This book begins with a discussion of the ways individual writers struggled against the expectation that they live out the culturally prescribed narrative of triumph. I follow with two chapters on how illness and disability damage a person's internal sense of self as well as sense of self over time. Finally, I focus on the efforts of people to give expression to the experiences of pain, disruption, and loss that characterize serious illness or injury. They consider the possibilities and limits of language, narrative form, and particular endings.

This book is not a survey of the literature on illness, although the literature is its evidence. Rather, it is an exploration of the nature of serious illness and the question of how one can speak or write about the pain, loss of self, and fear of death that so often go unarticulated. While this is a literary problem, it is first and foremost a philosophical and human problem. Those who have been pushed to the limits of their ability to cope know the difficulty of describing to others what they have been through. Schooled in suffering and articulate about written expression, the writers discussed here have something profound and radical to tell us about illness and narrative. They speak not out of a concern with techniques for managing illness but out of a deeply felt desire to describe their suffering and pain.

These writers create a literary space within which they acknowledge limitation and offer a range of views on the possibilities of writing in the face of death. Anatole Broyard powerfully endorses the notion that telling one's story is a way to stay alive even when dying. "To die is to be no longer human, to be dehumanized—and I think that language, speech, stories, or narratives are the most effective way to keep our humanity alive. To remain silent is literally to close down the shop of one's humanity."[40] While acknowledging the dissolution that is death, he believes in telling stories until death comes and suggests that, by choosing a style in which to be ill, a person can maintain his or her identity in the face of death. Harold Brodkey although writing in an attempt to remain himself in the face of his imminent death from AIDS, comes to a startling realization in *This Wild Darkness*—that the movement toward death is characterized by a progressive loss of identity that ultimately leaves him not only without the ability to tell a story, but without the ability to experience himself as ever having been a subject with a story to tell. "At times I cannot entirely believe I ever was alive, that I ever was another self, and wrote—and loved or failed to love. I do not really understand this erasure. Oh, I can comprehend a shutting down, a great power replacing me with someone else (and with silence), but this inability to have an identity in the face of death—I don't believe I ever saw this written about in all the death scenes I have read or in all the descriptions of old age."[41]

Others share with Brodkey this acknowledgment of the dissolution of the body and the self, what Murphy calls "the progressive and total destruction of my body, the reduction of all volition to quietude, the entombment of my mind in inert protoplasm."[42] By doing so they make room for the contemplation of mortality. Having resisted any coercion to view or approach their situation in a particular way, they acknowledge the ways illness or dying rob a person of the very identity with which he or she can make meaning or assert the self.

The question of language and its role in illness is at the heart of this book. From time immemorial writing has been a human act by which the mind mimics but also mediates its desire for immortality. It does this by fixing the voice on the page so that it survives even after the writer dies. In this sense writing is a defense against mortality. And in this sense, the story of writing is in itself a triumph narrative. The writers I will discuss demonstrate the deeply contradictory nature of this endeavor: within this form the culture has devised for creating permanence they discuss their own experience of impermanence.

These narratives, then, are characterized by a profound tension: their authors struggle to tell their story in order to stay alive and maintain their identity in the face of illness and dying, but they do so with the awareness that the very illness they describe can deprive them of their voice and self. They confront a fundamental paradox: Literature offers the possibility of representing the shattering experience of illness, but it proves woefully inadequate for depicting the nature of physical pain and the dissolution of the self. Nonetheless, in representing this failure of literature in the face of illness and death, these narratives prove indispensable: they capture something that is fundamental and generally unacknowledged—that the experience of illness and dying lies beyond our ability to describe it fully in language or to impart to it coherence or expressive form. Yet this very failure of literature paradoxically allows us as readers to approach the ground of desolation, where consolation will or will not come to each of us in our own time and in ways of our own making and unmaking.

— CHAPTER I —

The Cultural Story of Triumph

What the American public wants in the theater is tragedy with a happy ending.
—William Dean Howells (as reported in Edith
Wharton's introduction to *Age of Innocence*)

What harm can there be in a story of triumph? A person battles a disease, overcomes numerous obstacles, and, in the end, returns to life having learned some important lessons. If anything this story seems to offer hope, providing inspiration and a model for how to act in the face of serious illness or accident. No wonder people are captivated by these stories.

And yet not everyone feels so sanguine about triumph narratives. Some people find the triumph story at best a silly romance and at worst a cruel denial of their situation. After all, most people with a serious illness or injury are or have been in a state of emergency. They are struggling to come to terms with a terrifying diagnosis, serious damage to their body, or a future that feels shattered by the prospect of physical limitation or an early death. They may feel themselves unraveling or fear they will go crazy. While friends and relatives offer encouragement, they feel alone with their fears and preoccupied with the question of how they will cope. While the writers of triumph narratives may acknowledge this initial reaction to illness, they tend to gloss over the continuing difficulties of the experience and to write after the fact, imposing retrospectively a story of triumph.

Why not just ignore the story if it rings false? For one thing, most people have a complicated reaction: even if the triumph story rings false, it holds an attraction. It highlights those qualities we would all like to exhibit in the face of serious illness—an ability to fight against sickness and limitation, an optimism in the face of adversity. Embracing the triumph narrative also serves various psychological functions: it avoids the fact that suffering may serve no apparent purpose; it suggests that the progress of an illness leads in the direction of restored health; and it quells a person's anxiety over the possibility that his or her story may not have a happy ending.

It is also difficult to ignore a story that predominates in American culture and is widely insisted upon. In fact, the voices telling this story are so loud that they drown out others. The media bombard us with different variations on the triumph narrative. Advertisements pound home the notion that any bodily imperfection, or more accurately, any deviation from what is deemed the norm, can be overcome with procedures and products—plastic surgery, Botox, creams, lotions, and potions. When illness is depicted in TV ads for pharmaceuticals, people suffering the ailment not only appear more beautiful than the general population but also more vigorous. Television movies bathe the sufferer in soft light that hides the reality of the injured or suffering body.

As a culture we hide suffering. By keeping the ill, elderly, and dying out of view, we manage to keep the story of the damaged body, of physical weakness or limitation, out of earshot. When we do encounter the ill and disabled, we meet them with a coercive insistence that they rise above their suffering, battle their disease, and believe that everything will be fine in the end. We insist on optimism, put a spin on illness, and silence those who hurt, complain, or give up, labeling them "bad patients." We endlessly celebrate "survivors," while ignoring their equally valiant counterparts who did not survive. By subscribing so insistently to the narrative of triumph, we participate in a hysterical denial, as if by chanting "triumph" we can ward off mortality.

Often hospital customs and routines seem designed, whether intentionally or not, to keep the patient from telling a story different from that of triumph. Questions asked about the patient's medical history suggest a logical progression of events focused on symptoms, with little room for the patient's subjective experience. Technical medical terminology replaces an honest acknowledgment of the emotional toll serious illness and injury inflict. Some doctors, no more comfortable with illness than anyone else in our culture, avoid asking their patients how they feel. Or they themselves employ the vocabulary of triumph, assuring themselves the patient will recover. "We'll beat this together," they say. They may congratulate those who are "good patients"—that is, uncomplaining, strong, and brave. Because some insurance companies encourage doctors to see a fixed number of patients per hour, doctors may avoid asking open-ended questions in order to keep the encounter short.

Even those close to the sufferer suggest a triumph narrative when they talk about battling disease and remaining optimistic. Christina Middlebrook, disturbed to learn that the treatment she was given achieved a remission of more than a short duration only one-quarter of the time, relates her mother's response: "My mother tells me that I am not thinking right. She says that. Aloud. Over the phone. To me, her daughter. I am not thinking right! She tells me that I should focus on the percentage of patients who make it three years."[1] People feel discomforted by the ill person's expression of despair, so they offer stories of recoveries from serious illness—even if the recovery is from a different disease. The journalist Marjorie Williams, who died of liver cancer in 2005, describes her anger when "someone tried to cheer me up by reciting the happy tale of a sister-in-law's cousin who had liver cancer but now he's eighty and he hasn't been troubled by it in forty years. I wanted to scream, DON'T YOU KNOW HOW SICK I AM?"[2] Friends or relatives who tell this story are also members of a culture that denies illness and declines to honestly acknowledge sicknesses that are not readily overcome. They tell a story of survival in a desperate attempt to set things right, to reinstall denial. Meanwhile, the ill person who is told these stories is alone with the reality that recovery is not assured. As Williams, facing her own death, put it, "I felt abandoned, evaded, when someone insisted that I would live."[3]

Much of the brilliance of the play *Wit*, by Margaret Edson, lies in its depiction of the verbal exchanges between Vivian Bearing, the main character, and those caring for her. Bearing, a professor of English literature in the hospital with terminal ovarian cancer, is repeatedly called upon to live out the denial of death implicit in the triumph narrative. The play opens with Bearing saying to the audience, "Hi. How are you feeling today? Great. That's just great."

Mimicking the greeting of those who enter her room all day, she alerts the audience to the absurdity of this question, with its call for cheeriness in her dire situation. She goes on to say, "I have been asked 'How are you feeling today?' while I was throwing up into a plastic washbasin. I have been asked as I was emerging from a four-hour operation with a tube in every orifice, 'How are you feeling today?'" Finally, she states, "I am waiting for the moment when someone asks me this question and I am dead."[4]

Bearing's subjective emotional experience as well as her knowledge of what is happening to her body is irrelevant to most of those who treat her in the hospital. She is expected to answer "fine" to all inquiries about how she feels. Her complicated emotional reactions and the thoughts she communicates to the audience stand in bold contrast to the shallow and limited communication she engages in with her doctor. The play charts the ways the other characters do everything they can to deny her reality: they cut off serious conversation about dying, insist on a cheerful tone, and ignore her emotional suffering.

In American culture the narrative of triumph functions as a kind of myth: "a belief given uncritical acceptance by the members of a group especially in support of existing or traditional practices and institutions. . . . It is also used to designate a story, belief or notion commonly held to be true but utterly without factual basis."[5] The triumph narrative not only attempts to explain a phenomenon that is unknown and frightening—namely, illness and dying—but also embodies a belief that is given uncritical acceptance in our culture—that one can, with sufficient effort, triumph over illness. The literary scholar Anne Hunsaker Hawkins has explored the variety of templates that underlie stories of illness, including rebirth, battle, the journey, and "the myth of healthymindedness."[6] I use the term *triumph narrative* to refer primarily to the myth that those who are ill can confront their illness as a battle, do so with courage, and finally triumph and share with others the lessons they have learned.

As a concept the triumph narrative incorporates or makes reference to several predominant cultural myths—the Christian story that suggests salvation is a reward for suffering; the Horatio Alger myth whose moral is that people can, with hard work and determination, pull themselves up by their bootstraps; the New Age myth that implies illness can be controlled by proper behavior or attitude; and what I call the myth of the beautiful sufferer, which suggests that a person can remain beautiful even when terribly ill.

In the Christian story Jesus rises from the dead, and his body is restored to wholeness. Furthermore, his suffering results in redemption. While rarely used explicitly as a prototype for accounts of contemporary illness, the Christian story, with its depiction of triumph over physical suffering and of the restoration of the body to its former state, is often implicit in such narratives. It is the ultimate transformation story, bestowing meaning on experiences that might otherwise seem random and senseless; it offers hope and eternal life as an alternative to loss and despair; it places one imaginatively in the future and gives meaning to the experience of bodily pain. It also offers the comfort of expected resolution and a happy ending.

The Christian story is reflected in not only the content but also the shape of the triumph narrative. Barbara Ehrenreich, who writes political and social commentary, points out in "Welcome to Cancerland," which concerns her experience with breast cancer, that the shape of most personal memoirs is that of the religious narrative of the seventeenth century. "The personal narratives serve as testimonials and follow the same general arc as the confessional autobiographies required of seventeenth-century Puritans: first there is a crisis, often involving a sudden apprehension of mortality (the diagnosis or, in the old Puritan case, a stern word from on high); then comes a prolonged ordeal (the treatment or, in the religious case, internal struggle with the Devil); and finally, the blessed certainty of salvation, or its breast-cancer equivalent, survivorhood."[7]

Recognizing the dramatic appeal of the Resurrection as a prototype for his own illness story, Richard Seltzer, a retired surgeon who wrote about his Legionnaires' disease, adheres to the Christian story in his book *Raising the Dead* (a title that directly alludes to the Resurrection).[8] After twenty-four days in a coma, Seltzer is declared dead; all his vital signs indicate his body is no longer functioning. But ten minutes after that pronouncement, he takes a breath, sighs, and his vital signs return to normal. Toward the end of his book, Seltzer explains that he chose to frame the story of this anomalous physical event as a resurrection story because it would be dramatic. He realized that a story based solely on the notes he wrote after his hospital experience would lack "acceleration, crescendo, suspense and subtlety, irony, humor, the grotesque. . . . Most glaring is the absence of that single critical event that would raise the chronicle above the ordinary, a climax."9 For this reason he shapes his story as a resurrection. The climax occurs at the moment he seemed to stop breathing and then the plot unfolds from the point minutes later when his breathing resumes.

The triumph-over-illness narrative also contains echoes of the Horatio Alger myth. In the stories written by Horatio Alger the protagonist, by dint of hard work and moral rectitude, rises from poverty to achieve wealth and a place in society. In the triumph narrative the sufferer who works hard at recovery—rehabilitation, proper diet, rest—will be rewarded with survival or at least peace of mind. Here it is not suffering but work and determination that are rewarded by restored health. This distinctly American myth expresses a belief in progress toward a better future and in the efficacy of an optimistic attitude, what Harold Brodkey calls the "American fondness for the ad pitch . . . the forward-looking thing . . . swimming pools and corrective surgery."10 While the Horatio Alger myth is not referred to specifically by writers of illness memoirs, its celebration of the transformative value of hard work and determination underpins many narratives. When, for example, Hamilton Jordan ends his book with a list of suggestions for those who are ill, he implies that illness is a project that one must work hard at in order to succeed.

The New Age myth is evident in the writings of people like Norman Cousins, Bernie Siegel, Andrew Weil, and Deepak Chopra. Despite its cloak of spirituality the implications of this myth are actually quite harsh. There is no benign God who ultimately bestows salvation on those who suffer; rather, there is only the ill person who must be vigilant about vitamins, spirituality, and positive thinking. Because all responsibility for illness and its cure rests with the sufferer, failure to recover is blamed on the individual.

Many contemporary writers direct their wrath at this New Age myth for its oversimplification and hubris. Writing about his lover's dying of AIDS, Mark Doty suggests that New Age maxims, while perhaps appealing as a solution to life's difficulties, fall short in the end: "Take care of yourself, attune yourself to the inner life, rid yourself of negativity, focus on the light, and you'll be fine. But this seems to me, finally, a kind of kindergarten spirituality, a view of the soul written in broad crayon strokes."[11]

Some writers find gallows humor in the widespread cultural acceptance of the New Age myth. Marjorie Williams recounts that often she was asked a question about "what psychological affliction made me invite this cancer." With this in mind she hangs over her desk a *New Yorker* cartoon of two ducks in a pond. One of them is telling the other: "Maybe you should ask yourself why you're inviting all this duck hunting into your life right now."[12] Andrew Solomon in *The Noonday Demon* quotes a woman who felt he was just not trying hard enough to find a solution for his depression: "You might want to know that all the effects you describe come from chronic poisoning. Look around you. Did you have your home insecticided, your lawn herbicided? Are you living with particleboard subflooring? Until writers such as William Styron and yourself examine their surroundings for such exposures, and remove them, I have no patience with you and your depressive narratives."[13] Christopher Reeve, a quadriplegic as the result of a fall from a horse, noted that some New Age healers simply announce a cure when in fact there is none. Though skeptical, Reeve accepted the visit of one man from Ireland who worked on Reeve's upper body. When Reeve's arm moved spontaneously, as it tended to do randomly, this man declared, "The energy fields have been restored, allowing him to move."[14]

Reeve is a complicated figure. In public he was the ultimate embodiment of the triumph narrative, claiming that with enough effort a quadriplegic can reclaim some movement. Reeve did reclaim some movement, but it was minimal and the result of endless hours of physical therapy requiring the services of many professionals. While admired by many, Reeve still drew the ire of some disability activists who felt that by taking such a triumphalist position he glossed over the reality of paralysis. Another aspect of Reeve's story that generally goes unnoticed is that, at least early on in dealing with his paralysis and his future as a quadriplegic, he contemplated suicide.

The myth of the beautiful sufferer suggests that a person can remain physically beautiful even when ravaged by illness. Much nineteenth-century fiction includes a female character suffering from consumption who is depicted not as weakened and debilitated but as delicate, fragile, and beautiful in her dying; similarly the Romantic era poet John Keats is sentimentalized as sensitive and beautiful, not wasted, in his dying. In contemporary American culture this myth is given a different twist: however ill a person becomes, he or she is depicted as, or expected to remain, beautiful. Cosmetic companies offer free classes in makeup and hairstyling to women undergoing chemotherapy. People admire the "healthy glow" and thinness sometimes caused by treatments. If a women appears bald in public, she is seen as doing something radical, as if showing her actual physical state as a cancer patient represents an act of unseemly rebellion. This myth, with its denial of the reality of physical illness, embodies a deep antipathy toward bodily imperfection and a discomfort with the fact that illness makes people *look* sick. In a kind of psychological reaction formation, it substitutes a depiction of beauty when, in fact, what is feared is the damage illness can do to a person's appearance.

All of these varieties of the triumph myth represent a denial of the fact that illness often makes it impossible for a person to triumph, transcend, stay beautiful, or feel optimistic when suffering and a denial of the extent to which the difficulties of even an acute illness continue to reverberate throughout a life. While it may be soothing to hear that no problem is unsolvable, that we can affect the outcome of our illness by adopting a positive attitude, that we can remain beautiful, young, or vigorous no matter what the situation, a story that ignores the harsh reality of illness or disability does everyone a disservice. It lacks the complexity of real life. It keeps hidden how unmanageable certain aspects of illness are; it enables individuals and the culture to ignore the needs of the ill and disabled.

Polio as Triumph

Perhaps there is no better example of the clash in American culture between the reality of disease and the narrative of triumph than the story of polio victims in the 1950s. Charles Mee and Leonard Kriegel have each written poignantly and insightfully about their childhood experience with the disease. In *A Nearly Normal Life*, Mee, a playwright and writer, tells of how he and other children reacted to the 1950s' March of Dimes version of the triumph story and finally how he came to live and write his own alternative narrative.[15]

The March of Dimes campaign raised an astounding amount of money, enough to pay the expenses of anyone stricken with polio, as Mee points out. According to Mee, the campaign "got all mixed up with World War II and being a good American and believing in democracy and pitching in and winning."[16] The typical March of Dimes narrative depicted a child stricken by polio who, by virtue of the many dimes contributed by Americans, could walk on crutches across the stage, always with a smile on his face. At fund-raising events, still photographs or films would be shown that depicted "the child stricken with polio, the frightened parents rushing the child to the hospital, the child lying pale and emaciated in bed, near death. And then the lights would go up—and that very same child would be there in the banquet hall, making his triumphant way to the microphone, supported by a pair of crutches paid for by the March of Dimes."[17] Similarly, a March of Dimes poster "showed a boy before and after: with his head lolling in a neck brace, and then striding out robustly, with the legend 'Your dimes did this for me!'"[18]

Such stories were also planted by the publicity department of the National Foundation for Infantile Paralysis, the parent group for the March of Dimes, in magazines like *Reader's Digest*, according to Mee. An article in the *New York Times* Sunday magazine described cases of polio sufferers at Warm Springs, the rehabilitation hospital founded by FDR. "Take the case of a concert pianist whose hands were spared but whose feet were so affected that it was impossible for him to use the pedals of the piano. He has turned painter and his watercolors are bright and beautiful. That is the spirit of Warm Springs."[19] The story skips over the profound loss for the pianist of the use of his feet and moves on to celebrate his supposedly seamless transformation into a painter. Mee and the other children in the rehab hospital were skeptical of such stories. When they watched shows on television that depicted a triumphant return to health, they knew they were fiction. As Mee comments, "No one's experience of being seriously sick has ever been shown truly on television. No one's. Not once. I don't know why. . . . But the plot on television is always the same: Someone is struck by something; there is suffering; it is immensely sad; the stricken person is sad; the audience is made to empathize, pity, and cry; and then—very soon, before the burden of illness becomes too difficult—there is the full recovery, the happy, vigorous return to life itself, reaffirmation, optimism, victory. No child I knew at Sherman [Hospital] believed it."[20]

Mee points out two aspects of the triumph narrative that are problematic for the ill person: the story pays insufficient attention to the daily vicissitudes of bodily suffering, and it depicts a smooth, uninterrupted journey toward restored health or acceptance. The damage to victims of the disease, unless the case was a mild one, "alters their life, is knit into everything they do, shapes their careers and marriages and partnerships and relationships with their children." In addition, Mee argues, those who are disabled must recover over and over again throughout life—until they come to recognize "that damage is finally inescapable in life. . . . Their final coming to terms, their triumph, if it comes, always takes longer, is far more complicated, and is far more profound."[21]

Inescapable damage. No recovery. This is not a story most people want to hear. So for children with polio and their families it was the story that went unacknowledged. Doctors, therapists, and even parents often encouraged or even insisted that children with polio live out the triumph narrative, sometimes to the point of cruelty. Mee describes being placed in boiling tubs of water, swathed in hot, wet wool blankets that were then wrapped in plastic sheets for two or three hours, and having his limbs stretched. Although these treatments often did nothing to improve a child's ability to move his or her legs or hands, their uselessness went unacknowledged even by the children undergoing them. Perhaps these children feared disappointing their parents and caregivers, or perhaps they had no other narrative available to them.

These physical ordeals bear an uncanny resemblance to those depicted in religious narratives. Given that it must have been apparent to doctors and parents that these treatments did not increase movement in the children's limbs, the suffering they caused may actually have contributed to the continuance of the treatments. If suffering is the prerequisite for redemption in the Christian triumph narrative, perhaps people believed one must suffer to get better. Or perhaps it was simply too painful to imagine that the suffering of these children was for nought.

Like most children with polio, Mee accepted the treatments and physical therapy as part of what was required, either out of hope for improvement or as proof that he was not accepting defeat. He agreed to have one operation, for example, not because he thought it would help (many such operations had already failed) but because his parents and doctors so wanted him to have it, as a last resort. After the surgery, Mee accompanied his doctor to a class where the doctor presented him as a kind of specimen to his medical students. There Mee testified to an improvement in his functioning, even though he felt none. Finally, when he could take the charade no longer, Mee spoke out: "No, I don't think it has made any difference at all, really; maybe I'm a *little* worse."[22] He was not invited back.

In his discussion of occupational therapy for the disabled, Mee notes an essential contradiction in our attitudes, represented in two conflicting narratives promoted about disability. On the one hand, the protagonist of the triumph narrative is self-sufficient, enterprising, and successful in overcoming adversity. This narrative features "a person who makes every possible effort to regain an independent self-supporting life for himself, who, against great odds, works at a job we find surprising a handicapped person is able to perform, makes a successful career, never mentions his disability, never betrays any suggestion of self-pity."[23] On the other hand, another narrative was suggested to children who were disabled, that of a life in a sheltered workshop where they would perform menial tasks without ever being given the opportunity to have a more fulfilling work life. One time Mee wheeled in his chair into a room where he saw children with polio and older people with strokes hunched in their wheelchairs, "learning to perform tasks that would help them to lead independent lives: weaving baskets, punching holes in leather belts, making a macramé key chain." His reaction was stark: "I don't think I ever saw anything more alarming."[24]

While Mee struggled not to scorn the efforts of the people in that room, he explains that he needed to reject the narrative implied in their activity—that physical limitation closes the door on the possibility of creative work. "The sheer terror of coming so close to having such limited abilities for the rest of my life triggered some deep inner voice to yell at me to run," he says.[25] His ultimate refusal to participate in occupational therapy, which for him was a refusal to submit to a life of deadening activity, was viewed by those around him as resistance, as a form of depression or failure to adjust. In fact, Mee's refusal allowed him to look for and ultimately find a satisfying life as a teacher and writer.

Neither of the two narratives available to those who are disabled is adequate. The first, that bodily damage can be overcome by anyone who has sufficient determination and optimism, is not true to life. Many children who had polio never walked, despite enormous effort on their part. The second, that illness or accident simply renders one incapable of any but rote tasks, is also false. It relegates the disabled to sheltered workshops where they do mindless work even if they retain great mental capacity. These opposing narratives reflect the cultural inability to deal with illness except in extreme terms—either to deny the damage of polio completely or to see only the damage and then give up hope of a fulfilling life for those who are disabled.

Mee does not simply reject the triumph narrative but realizes that its appeal resides in the fact that people, including the disabled, cannot bear failure. He understands that people need to embrace stories of triumph and ignore stories of people who do not get better. "If a girl spends her life in an iron lung, we want to hear how she triumphed over it, how she became a deeper, better, wiser, more profoundly philosophical and transcendent person for it; how, in fact, it was almost a wonderful advantage to spend a life in an iron lung, because of the insight it yielded."[26] He goes on to say, "We don't need to learn how to fail in our lives; we need to learn how to succeed. . . . We want to rehearse success; we want to know what qualities of character are needed for triumph."[27] In the end, however, Mee focuses on the personal and societal problems that result from this "refusal to recognize the possibility of failure, the refusal to accept the tragic nature of life."[28] For a boy with polio this refusal had very personal ramifications. "This culture made me feel, as a boy, that I needed to keep my chin up, reassure my parents about how well I was doing, never be sad, look to the future, be optimistic. . . . It made me live a lie, confuse myself about who I was and what I felt and how life was for me."[29]

Mee's critique of cultural attitudes toward disability is part of his larger critique of American culture and its insistence on triumph as a way to deny certain realities—that not every one in our society succeeds in escaping poverty, that death does occur, that not all problems can be fixed. He sees the triumph narrative as complicitous in the creation of an America "where a vast network of institutions has been built to hide the millions who cannot pull themselves up by their bootstraps . . . where death is denied, where we undertake extravagant attempts to fix the unfixable in hospital operating rooms and in sovereign countries such as Vietnam."[30]

Leonard Kriegel, a retired professor of American literature at City College of New York who had polio when he was eleven, also recognizes the extent to which dominant cultural myths affected his development and reaction to polio.[31] Kriegel focuses on the coming-of-age myths available to an American boy, particularly that personified by Tom Sawyer. For Kriegel Tom Sawyer resonated with his own wish as a boy, and later as an adult, to use his imagination to run away and, in his case, escape his crippled state and imagine himself whole. Kriegel describes how at age eleven he was unable (or more likely, he suggests, refused) to learn from his physical therapist how to go with a fall in order to avoid injuring himself. Day after day he would dutifully perform all the expected components of the technique: he learned to throw his legs from his hip and dangle from the parallel bars. But when his physical therapist told him to fall on the mat, he couldn't do it. He felt rage and humiliation at his inability, but he came to wonder if perhaps he "had unconsciously seized upon some fundamental resistance to the forces that threatened to overwhelm me."[32] After a month of terror and shame he was able to master the fall, a fact that he understood as a willingness to accept his situation and not run away.

In an essay entitled "Taking It"[33] Kriegel recognizes as well the importance of another myth available to American boys—that to be a man is to hold your ground and endure without complaint whatever hardship life bestows. On the positive side this myth inspired Kriegel to defy physical limits: he walked miles, did hundreds of push-ups, worked out until he collapsed. He was taking it like a man. Many men with disabilities, including Mee, describe living out this kind of physical triumph. For example, Stephen Kuusisto, the poet and educator who wrote *Planet of the Blind*, describes working out for hours, becoming strong as a way to compensate for his limited sight and as a personal challenge.[34] Kriegel came to view this myth as representing not so much a mature acceptance of life, as a kind of macho endurance resulting in further damage to his body. He believes that the physical exercise he performed to compensate for physical limitation actually left him with the arthritis he suffers as an older man.[35]

Kriegel highlights two predominant representations of the disabled in American literature. The "charity cripple" is the person who accepts his or her situation, is not demanding, and becomes the recipient of the largess of others. An example is Tiny Tim in Charles Dickens's *A Christmas Carol*. The second representation is that of the "demonic cripple," whose refusal to accept his situation warps his personality. In literature the "demonic cripple" inspires fear because others cannot understand what drives his pursuit of vengeance. He "is consumed by an isolation that goes beyond accident to harden into the very center of his existence."[36] As an example Kriegel points to Shakespeare's character Richard III. For Kriegel these one-dimensional and extreme depictions are problematic because they come to define a person from the outside. "In what we call literature, as well as in popular culture, we are what others make of us."[37] Kriegel claims that in accepting others' definitions of disability, "what we invariably discover is that our true selves, our own inner lives, have been auctioned off so that we can be palatable rather than real."[38] A child who accepts himself as an object for the charity of others becomes by definition dependent. "Only a considerable act of defiance can possibly save that child from the fate of being permanently dependent."[39]

As an example of that defiance Kriegel describes a boy he glimpsed in the isolation room of the hospital where Kriegel stayed. "His back was naked and I could see the outline of every bone ripped with bedsores and blisters, and raw blotches of skin."[40] The nurse, of whose charity the boy was the unwilling recipient, said of him, "I've never known a more obstinate boy." She went on, "Never said a word. Not to anyone. You'd think a boy like that would pray. But it was just silence in that room."[41] Kriegel sees the boy's silence and refusal to be polite, compliant, and grateful as "a way of resisting, of refusing to be swallowed up by the accidental evil of an indifferent universe."[42] Even as a child Kriegel believed that this boy's resistance was an assertion of self. "I admired him. I admired him as much as I have ever admired anyone."[43]

Mee and Kriegel offer subtle, complex depictions of the way negative ideas about disability played out in their lives and their fight against the adoption of the culture's depiction of them. Each came up against a culture that expected of them a particular story: that they accept their situation, work hard to recover, appreciate the efforts of others, and ultimately, triumph, at least in spirit, over the damage to their bodies. To accept the role designated for them by their culture, they argue, would have been to deny their rage, impotence, and fear, and thus to betray themselves. In the end they tell their own stories, in which they develop a different view of what constitutes triumph: that they face reality and then move beyond their physical limitations, not by denying the damage or disease but by finding a way to live a full life despite being cognizant of that damage. By choosing careers where their physical disabilities do not hinder them, they are able to live outside their limitations.

Triumph as Hindrance

Those who are almost totally blind have a complex relationship to the triumph narrative. By dint of enormous effort they are often able to function normally—at least apparently. And yet some come to believe this kind of triumph and adaptation come at too great a cost. Stephen Kuusisto and Georgina Kleege, two authors who are blind, describe how they spent a major portion of their lives living out the culturally proscribed narrative of triumph only to discover later that, in fact, their apparent success actually deprived them of the very tools that would have helped them cope better with their blindness and, paradoxically, would have made them more independent. Stephen

Kuusisto has been legally blind from the time of his birth. Although he can see only colors and shapes "like a kaleidoscope," through extraordinary effort he became so adept at reading clues that he could often pass as sighted. He managed to ride a bicycle and go jogging; he read books by holding them close to his face; he declined, as a matter of pride, the use of mechanical aids, cane, or guard dog, and in so doing he lived out the culture's story—that given determination he could ignore physical limitation and function normally. His mother, colluding in his denial, perhaps in an attempt to keep him from being marginalized or labeled as inferior, rejected a special school for him. She simply would not "give in to" his blindness or his need to learn Braille or use a cane. As a boy, Kuusisto was busy keeping to himself how little he could see. "I thrived on suborning my blindness. My parents were perfect accomplices, loving, eccentric, well-meaning, dotty."[44]

Not until he was enrolled at the University of Iowa did he accept the limitations his blindness imposed on him. When he applied for Social Security assistance, the blind advisor assigned to him discerned the extent to which Kuusisto denied his blindness. He introduced him to a special tape recorder and a high-resolution camera that could scan a page and produce the text in large print on a screen, and he suggested readers and books on tape. He insisted that Kuusisto stop riding his bike. He explained that Kuusisto's well-meaning parents had not been able to deal with his blindness in any way but denial. He suggested, "The cane is about being alive. It serves all kinds of functions. . . . You spend a lot less time explaining yourself."[45]

The counselor's advice echoes the point both Mee and Kriegel came to make—that the denial inherent in trying to live out the triumph narrative actually prevents one from living a fuller life. Nonetheless, Kuusisto declined the advisor's proffered aid and continued his performance, living as if he could see better than he did. Only when a cut on his good reading eye left him completely unable to see for a time did he finally accept his blindness and, as he explains, give up his commitment to living out a triumph narrative. "Until the accident, I imagined myself as a romantic figure, the poet who is nearly blind, the one who requires only a table, a little light, and some silence. In this vision I was heroic."[46] He goes on to describe the daring and, in fact, reckless and grandiose behaviors in which he had engaged. "I'd learned to travel alone in the world even though I couldn't read street signs or the intricate maps in transit systems. I went skiing, played pick-up basketball with the international students at the University of Helsinki even though I couldn't see the fast-moving ball or the hoop."[47]

On the surface Kuusisto, by ignoring his blindness and taking on so many challenges, looked successful. He managed to live in a manner worthy of the best triumph narrative. But by accepting the cultural premium placed on looking "normal," he never really examined whether his choices were best for him. In the end he came to realize not only that denial of his blindness was crazy and irresponsible—he repeatedly put himself and others in danger—but that it was also exhausting and limiting. He had to work very hard at activities like reading and walking that could have been made much easier had he used Braille, a seeing eye dog, and a cane. But to accept those aids, he had to give up the fantasy that success meant denying his physical limitations.

Georgina Kleege, a novelist, essayist, and translator who wrote *Sight Unseen*, similarly defined her life as a seeing person who was visually impaired, not as a blind person.[48] Kleege was pronounced blind in 1967 when she was eleven. Because she held books close to her eyes to read, it was assumed she was near-sighted. When tests indicated this was not the case, her ophthalmologist concluded she was faking and pursued the matter no further. Eventually additional tests indicated she suffered from macular degeneration, a disease that was causing her to slowly lose sight. She was told there was no cure and was sent off "with no glasses, no advice, no explanations."[49] When she asked about learning Braille, she was told it was unnecessary and too hard. Perhaps the triumph narrative played a role here. If she could manage to read without Braille, she could appear normal. In fact, she was ingenious about finding ways to adapt: she read with magnifying glasses and held the book close to her face. This caused pain above her eye that spread to her forehead and other eye and also caused pain in her neck and shoulder muscles.

Like Kuusisto, she came to the realization that living as "normal" was not so much a triumph as an unnecessary struggle; by denying limits, she actually struggled more than would have been necessary. Kleege's experience in writing her book has a particularly dramatic aspect. She set out to write a book about cultural representations of blindness in language, film, and literature, about the phenomenology of blindness, about attempts to capture in words the visual experience of someone with impaired sight, and finally, about reading, an activity central to her identity. In the process, however, she comes to understand how little she was able to see compared to other people. As a result, she came to identify herself as blind and began to use Braille and a cane. Kleege came to understand that, in addition to causing her headaches, her denial of her blindness left her far more dependent on others for help than she would have been had she adjusted to using aids and learning Braille. It was with considerable difficulty and in the face of continued resistance from those around her that she eventually taught herself Braille. Her journey is really about her success in rejecting the cultural narrative and choosing instead a narrative that acknowledges limitation and lays the groundwork for better ways to cope.

Sometimes insistence on triumph results in unnecessary emotional suffering. In *A Leg to Stand On* Oliver Sacks, the neurologist famous for his writing and explorations of neurological states, describes his experience in the hospital after seriously injuring his leg while running from a bull he encountered on a mountain in Norway.[50] After a leg surgery considered successful by his doctors, Sacks found himself experiencing not what he was told to expect—some atrophy in his leg—but rather complete atrophy. Unable to produce a response in his limp leg, Sacks felt an increasing panic. He waited eagerly for his surgeon, Dr. Swan, to arrive, needing from him "the voice, the simplicity, the conviction, of authority. 'Yes, I understand. It happens. Don't fret. Do this! Believe me! You will soon be well.'"[51] While Sacks realized the surgeon might not be able to offer such reassurance, he still looked forward to an honest and understanding response. If the doctor said, "Sacks, it's the damnedest thing—I don't know what you've got. But we'll do our best to find out," Sacks would respect that. "I should respect whatever he said so long as it was frank and showed respect for me, for my dignity as a man."[52]

Sacks describes Dr. Swan's arrival as a religious procession. The staff's bustling preparation for that arrival produced "extraordinary stillness." The surgeon appeared, "accompanied by Sister bearing his surgical and ceremonial tools on a tray" and followed by a retinue of other doctors and students. Despite all the pomp and circumstance, "Swan neither looked at me nor greeted me, but took the chart which hung at the foot of my bed and looked at it closely." He was pleased that Sacks reported that his leg was fine "surgically speaking."[53] But when Sacks reported that he could not contract the quadriceps of his leg, Swan replied "sharply and decisively" that there was nothing wrong with the leg. When Sacks tried to object, Swan "held up his hand, like a policeman halting traffic"[54] and brusquely left the room. Swan refused to allow his patient, Sacks, to undermine his conclusion that the surgery was a success.

In this conflict over the nature of the story to be told, Swan insists on triumph. Sacks, realizing how seriously this encounter had dashed his hopes of being understood, told himself that the formality of grand rounds demanded the doctor play the role of "All-knowing Specialist" and he that of "Know-nothing Patient." Sacks then tried to explain his situation to the registrar, another doctor, who impatiently dismissed Sacks's complaints as "vague and subjective." The registrar said, "We orthopods are really carpenters, in a way. We are called in to do a job. We do it and that's that."[55] Only years later, after nerve conduction tests and electromyograms, did Sacks have the objective evidence of physical damage.[56] Sacks had hoped the understanding of his doctor would serve as bulwark against his increasing fears, but "by saying nothing . . . he took away a foothold, the human foothold, I so desperately needed."[57] Sacks describes the abyss of despair he sank into, feeling he was losing himself. He believes that his doctor could have helped him, that human communication can function to make psychic survival possible even in the face of overwhelming terror at the loss of self. Instead, his doctor's coldness and refusal to listen to Sacks's less triumphant story left him in a state of psychic disintegration.

Depression, a disease whose severity is often underestimated, is one in which the patient's narrative is often rejected. Like Sacks, who believed his experience with Dr. Swan precipitated a depression,

Andrew Solomon asserts that an experience in the emergency room precipitated his third mental breakdown. Arriving after he slipped on the stairs and dislocated his shoulder, he tried to explain to the staff that he needed them to treat his pain immediately because untreated physical pain from an attack of kidney stones had precipitated a previous depressive episode. The staff told him to stop complaining—that dislocated shoulders are painful until they are put back in place; he should exercise self-control and pull himself together. When he again explained that he was not so afraid of the pain as he was worried about psychiatric complications, he was told that he was "being 'childish' and 'uncooperative.'"[58] Not until four and a half hours after his arrival did he finally receive what he calls "some meaningful pain relief."[59]

During the three days after this episode Solomon had acute suicidal feelings of a kind he had not experienced since his first breakdown. He cried all the time and found tasks like answering the telephone and putting on his socks overwhelming. Many suicides occur because of such failures to recognize the seriousness of depression, Solomon suggests. The true narrative of depression—that a person cannot function—flies in the face of the American belief in optimism and taking charge. A person who cannot function is easily viewed as having a weakness of character, not a disease, sometimes with disastrous consequences for the sufferer.

The Internalized Story of Triumph

Finally, those who are ill confront the triumph narrative not only in their culture but also in themselves. They have internalized this narrative that so predominates in our culture. Nancy Mairs explains that as a disabled adult she feels a certain pressure to live out the triumph myth by ascribing to the notion that disability can be managed and limitations overcome. One evening she received a phone call before dinner from a college student who read her essay "On Being a Cripple" and called because she thought she had MS. Mairs explained that she was sitting down to dinner with her family but spoke to the young woman briefly. Later she wondered if she should have gotten the girl's number and called her back to talk more. But then Mairs thought, "What am I supposed to do about Jennifer? Take away her MS, if that indeed is what she has? Failing that, calm her fears? Give her a college degree? Transform her husband, who will almost certainly leave her, and sooner rather than later, from a scared kid into a pillar of support and sympathy? I may wish I were God, but the truth is that I can't even tie my own shoes."[60]

Mairs catches herself being drawn into the role of the older, wiser woman with MS who is living out the triumph myth by rising above her illness and helping others to do the same. She feels, on the one hand, that she should offer the comfort the myth provides for: illness is unfortunate but one can rise above it. On the other hand she knows the truth is far different: most likely MS will wreak devastation on this girl's life: probably there is little that can be done about Jennifer's disease; her family will be strained beyond imagining; and there will be little easy comfort for her.

Elsewhere Mairs catches herself subscribing to another, more negative narrative—one that portrays the disabled as deserving of charity, as inferior. While sitting in a café Mairs notices an attractive women lunching with a man. Her first thought is that she is flirting with him. But upon leaving the restaurant Mairs notices the woman's wheelchair and immediately imagines a different scenario. "Oh, the poor thing!" How courageous she is to fix herself up and get out of the house on a day as hot as this. And what a thoughtful man—her brother, it must be—treating her to lunch to cheer her up."[61]

Mairs explains that when she was initially diagnosed with MS she "subscribed to the major social myths about the disabled woman."[62] She worried that she would be considered undesirable and never achieve success in life. She wondered, "Could I go on teaching, and if so, would anybody want to hire me? Would my husband still find me sexually attractive, and could he accept my increasing need for help? Would my children resent having a mother who couldn't do everything the other mothers could? How would I survive if they all abandoned me?"[63]

The triumph narrative holds enormous sway in our culture. It is not simply a narrative that one can take or leave, but one that the ill and disabled must contend with in the media, in personal interactions with doctors, in conversations with friends and family, and even in themselves. Often this narrative is invoked as a way to cover up more negative attitudes toward those who are ill or disabled—that they are actually less capable than others. Because the triumph story has become so embedded in our culture, its repercussions play out with regard to individual patients. Children with polio are expected to walk; those who are blind are encouraged to function as if they can see. It is a narrative that most of us have internalized. As a result, we not only expect others to remain optimistic and transcend illness or accident, but when we ourselves are ill or disabled, we struggle to live up to this impossible ideal. When we cannot find it in ourselves to battle, to look healthy, to remain optimistic, we feel we are failing. It is also a narrative whose denial of limitation and death has a destructive impact on large groups of people. Those who cannot triumph are looked down upon; the needs of the disabled are not adequately addressed; and the dying are often not allowed to die before being subjected to high-tech interventions.

Although the writers I have cited argue for an alternative to the triumph narrative that acknowledges the reality of both physical and emotional suffering, the fact is that most of us do not have an alternative way of conceptualizing our experience. We tend to tell our story in the form of a triumph narrative. As Arthur Frank puts it so well, "The shape of the telling is molded by all the rhetorical expectations that the storyteller has been internalizing ever since he first heard some relative describe an illness, or she saw her first television commercial for a non-prescription remedy, or he was instructed to 'tell the doctor what hurts' and had to figure out *what* counted as the story that the doctor wanted to hear. From their families and friends, from the popular culture that surrounds them, and from the stories of other ill people, storytellers have learned formal structures of narrative, conventional metaphors and imagery, and standards of what is and is not appropriate to tell."[64] The writers I will discuss attempt to free themselves from the confines of the triumph narrative to tell a story that focuses more directly on their own emotional experience.

Arthur Kleinman in *The Illness Narratives* notes the importance of this different approach to the story of illness. He relates an experience from his early days as a medical student, when he was asked to hold the hand of a badly burned seven-year-old girl who screamed throughout the daily removal of dead tissue from her body.[65] He repeatedly tried to distract her and bring her back to her normal life by asking about her family and school. His efforts failed completely. Only when he asked how she tolerated her treatment and what it was like for her did she stop screaming and talk directly to him, describing the painful, daily ritual. In many ways the triumph narrative functions as a distraction, a way to bring the ill and all of us back to thoughts of "normal" life. Narratives that describe the actual felt experience of those who are ill or injured do something different. They allow those who are ill to speak honestly about their suffering. They allow those who listen to come closer to understanding that suffering. And, in the end, there is nothing more compelling.

— CHAPTER II —

Character: The Damaged Self

*The unexpected failure of the body is a shocking catastrophe
that threatens the flimsy edifice we call the "self."*
—Robert McCrum, *My Year Off*

In *The Noonday Demon* Andrew Solomon offers this description of the collapse of self that characterized his depression:

> Shortly before my thirty-first birthday, I went to pieces. My whole system seemed to be caving in. . . . On the way home from the store, I suddenly lost control of my lower intestine and soiled myself. I could feel the stain spreading as I hastened home. . . . I did not sleep much that night, and I could not get up the following day. . . . I moved my tongue but there were no sounds. I had forgotten how to talk. Then I began to cry, but there were no tears, only a heaving incoherence. I was on my back. I wanted to turn over, but I couldn't remember how to do that either. I tried to think about it but the task seemed colossal.[1]

Solomon is describing the near total inability to function that characterized his emotional collapse. This experience of some degree of disintegration of the self is often characteristic of the experience of serious physical illness or injury as well. Robert Lipsyte describes the kind of physical breakdown that accompanied his knowledge that he had a life-threatening illness. In his case the disease was testicular cancer, the thought of which could produce in him at any time the reaction he calls "The Dread." He explains: "In my case, the symptoms of The Dread were dry mouth, loose bowels, a toothache in my gut, worst of all numbness, a physical and psychic paralysis that could strap me to a chair for hours, thoughtless, staring."[2] Max Lerner describes his initial experience of his cancer diagnosis in similar terms: "I felt the shock deep in my offending guts. Suddenly I had lost my center of gravity, which depended on my belief in my body as a given, a habitation for my 'self.'"[3] Robert Murphy, the anthropologist who had a tumor of the spinal column that caused a progression to quadriplegia, points out how central to a person's sense of self are the bodies and the organs that enable one to breathe, eat, see, and hear: "These organs, and the body itself, are among the foundations upon which we build our sense of who and what we are."[4]

While the nature and degree of damage in different illnesses and disabilities vary widely, all serious illness and disability share this fundamental characteristic: damage to the body constitutes damage to the self. On one end of the spectrum is the diminished sense of self that accompanies a mundane illness like the flu or the temporary disability caused by a broken leg. The sufferer temporarily feels out of sorts, distracted by the body's discomfort, preoccupied, not quite himself or herself. In the middle of the spectrum are those illnesses or accidents one survives but which involve some significant—whether temporary or permanent—change in the body and consequent loss of function. In these instances a person's sense of a stable self may be profoundly damaged. The self is often experienced as divided. The body or the affected body part is experienced as alien; in order to preserve the integrity of the self, the person may disown the offending body part. In situations where pain is all-consuming, the self is also severely compromised. Because the person in serious pain generally turns inward and withdraws from life, he or she loses not a particular function but the overall ability to function. Intense pain preoccupies the sufferer; it sucks up all available energy. The pained self becomes the only self. Finally, at the far end of the spectrum is the total loss of self one experiences when near death—what Harold Brodkey refers to as the "inability to have an identity in the face of death."[5]

In *A Whole New Life* Reynolds Price explores the notion that serious illness and disability are actually catastrophic. He tells us that the "Greek word *catastrophe* means an *overturning*, an *upending*—a system disarranged past reassembly, all signals reversed." He states that the "list of common catastrophes that wait for a final chance at each of us is virtually endless. . . . Birth disasters, unstoppable cancers, disorders of the blood and lymph, external wounds to flesh and bone, those devastations in which the body turns on itself and eats its own substance, the mind's estrangement, the still irreparable disconnection of electrical service to major parts."[6] All those who write narratives about such kinds of experiences are attempting to represent and make sense of their impact on the self. But they do so in radically different ways.

Those who write a triumph narrative, even while depicting the devastating events of illness or accident, tend to represent the self as stable and robust and therefore able to battle disease and maintain a positive attitude while doing so. They posit an internal intact self that remains strong even in the face of the most devastating events and a self that remains continuous over time. In doing so, I would argue, they minimize the extent to which serious illness or accident severely destabilizes the very self so badly needed to cope with disease and limitation. Told retrospectively, the triumph narrative views the events of illness in light of a person's recovery or return to life.

Narratives that describe the devastation of serious illness or disability focus less on the final resolution than on the actual experience of the self in the aftermath of illness or injury. It is not that their authors fail to recover, survive, or even triumph, but their achievement rests in acknowledging all aspects of their experience—including the shattering of the self and the upending of their life. Rather than describe a self that remains intact whatever the assault on the body, these writers suggest a fragile self fending off disintegration. Some depict a self that is damaged, diminished, or collapsed. Others demonstrate the intricate ways those suffering physical trauma preserve the fragile self by disowning the body or the body's experience. Finally, some describe the way they repudiate aspects of their own experience that, if fully felt, might simply overwhelm them.

The Triumphant, Resilient Self

The notion that the self can be resilient under any circumstances is enormously appealing. We are moved and reassured when a person who loses use of his or her legs manages to live a full life, when someone who becomes blind writes a book, travels, or lives a "normal" life.

Perhaps the idea of resilience is so powerful because the alternative—a self that can be compromised, overwhelmed, or broken—is so threatening to contemplate. And yet, we can wonder, is the representation of the ill or disabled self as intact an accurate one, or is it designed to protect us from the real frailty of our sense of self? Nancy Smith, in an article about the writing of Primo Levi, the Italian chemist, writer, and survivor of Auschwitz, questions the notion that the self can remain resilient in situations of extreme stress.[7] While her focus is on the Holocaust, her observations have relevance to serious illness.

Noting that the story of survivors of the Holocaust is often framed as one of triumph, she looks at Levi's writing to emphasize the complicated reality of their situation. While the arrival at the end of World War II of the Russians at Auschwitz and the defeat of the Germans was certainly a political and military victory, framing the overall story as triumph, in Smith's view, distorts the reality of what it was like for the nearly thousand sick and dying inmates left behind by the Nazis. She quotes Levi: "ragged, decrepit, skeleton like patients . . . no longer in control of their own bowels, they have fouled everywhere. . . . Other starving specters like ourselves wandered around searching, unshaven, with hollow eyes, greyish skeleton bones in rags, shaky on their legs."[8] Smith understands Levi to be saying that "what we are witnessing here is *not* the precious resilience of the human spirit. It is rather the horrible collapse of the human spirit." She goes on to say, "Do not be deceived. These Nazi camps were masterfully designed to be resiliency-killing factories, which systematically shattered every ounce of the human psyche so there would be no bouncing back."[9]

When people tell the story of serious illness and disability as triumph, they are adhering to a belief that the human spirit can remain resilient even under the most extreme conditions. In so doing they minimize the damage done to the self by excruciating pain, toxic treatments, and the loss of basic functions. Generally the triumph narrative is told retrospectively with a view to underlining the attitudes and behavior that produced the triumph—faith in God, a fighting spirit, an optimistic attitude. The movement of the plot is inevitably toward a return to life as normal. Implicit in its representation is the notion that the self has remained intact and resilient enough to meet the challenge posed by illness and that in the end the self is restored to its former state. While many who are ill or disabled display enormous reserves of strength, an insistence on resiliency often becomes a way to ignore the devastation and even collapse endured by many.

Those who tell the story of illness or injury as it is experienced often present a far more radical picture of the damage done to the self as perceived both internally and across time. Recognizing the absurdity of expecting resiliency of a person in extreme distress, they demonstrate how those who lose the ability to walk or see are absorbed with the loss and the enormity of the adjustment they face. These writers represent the internal self not as intact and resilient but as at best disrupted and at worst shattered. They depict the self perceived over time not as continuous but so altered as to seem an entirely different self. These writers stress that serious illness and accident do not simply affect the body, leaving the self intact to rise up like some noble warrior beside the fallen brother soldier, the body, as the triumph narrative would have it. They see the body and the self as one; this means that they fall as one.

The title of Susanna Kaysen's book—*Girl Interrupted*—captures the dual impact of illness on the internal self and the self in time.[10] Kaysen writes the story of her emotional breakdown from depression at the age of eighteen, which interrupted her life as a college student. But her title suggests that her illness also interrupted her sense of an ongoing, intact self—the *girl*. In this chapter I will consider the damage to the internal self as it is represented in various narratives of serious illness and disability and in the next chapter the impact of illness or injury on the self over time.

The Damaged Self

Whether damage to the body results from illness or accident, the experience of damage to the self is similar. In both situations physical damage restricts a person's functioning, dominates thought, and profoundly alters the experience of self. Robert Murphy,[11] whose movement toward quadriplegia involved a progressive loss of function, concluded from his own experience and observations of others that the "four most far-reaching changes in the consciousness of the disabled are: lowered self-esteem; the invasion or occupation of thought by physical deficits; a strong undercurrent of anger; and the acquisition of a new, total, and undesirable identity."[12] It's not simply that people have a *different* experience of self, Murphy is saying, but they acquire an identity they do not want and probably do not like.

The novelist and editor Robert McCrum makes a similar point about the kind of damage to the self that can occur. McCrum suffered a stroke at the age of forty-two.[13] In *My Year Off* he tells how the effects of his stroke reverberated through every aspect of his self and life. Because his stroke damaged functions central to his identity, it called into question that very identity. Although his vocal cords remained intact, the injury to his brain left him without the ability to find words or enunciate them in normal order. "The failure of articulation seemed such a fundamental failure, and one that went to the core of my self-esteem,"[14] McCrum said. His stroke shattered his confidence and more generally his understanding of who he was. "It is an event that goes to the core of who and what you are, the Youness of you. First of all, the event happens in your brain which is, without becoming unduly philosophical, the command centre of the self. Your brain is you: your moods, your skills, your character, your intelligence, your emotions, your self-expression, your self."[15]

The point these writers are making is that the story of serious illness or accident is not primarily one of resilience. While they tell the story of how people deal with damage to the body and the self, they do something more—they underline, each step of the way, what has been lost and will never be recovered even as they find a way to deal with the damage that has been done to body and psyche. The catastrophic event is not something the effects of which can be confined to the past but something that continues to define and have repercussions for the self. As Lucy Grealy suggests in the title of her book *Autobiography of a Face*, the story of her life—her autobiography—is the same as the story of her face, damaged by repeated surgeries for a childhood cancer.[16]

The Disembodied Self

When damage to the body results in a loss of function, many people report that the affected body part seems alien, as if the injured arm or leg no longer belongs to the body. McCrum describes his own experience of disembodiment after his stroke. "I was puzzled and curious. It was almost as though I was not in my body, the body that seemed to have let me down so badly. (I still wonder if the 'I' who is typing this with my 'good' right hand, is the same as the 'I' who used to peck away, two-handed, at 50 w.p.m.)."[17] Later he notices that he talks about his leg differently depending on whether he can move it or not. "When it was immobilized it was always 'the'; only when movement came back did I claim it as 'my.'"[18] It is as if the immobilized body part is dead and the part of the self connected to that nonfunctioning part is also dead.

Oliver Sacks offers a profound philosophical reflection on the intricate intertwining of perceptions of body and self. After his surgery Sacks began to realize that his inability to move the muscle in his leg represents a more fundamental breakdown of the essential components of his self. This realization upsets him even more than the idea of a paralyzed muscle. "What seemed, at first, to be no more than a local, peripheral breakage and breakdown now showed itself in a different, and quite terrible, light—as a breakdown of memory, of thinking, of will—*not just a lesion in my muscle, but a lesion in me.*"[19] Like others who find part of their body to be alien and inanimate, he came to feel that his immovable leg bore "no relation whatever to me. It was absolutely *not-me.*" Later he calls it "a ludicrous object with no relation to me"[20] and realizes that although the leg still exists, he no longer has a subjective experience of it. He has "lost the inner image, or representation, of the leg. There was a disturbance, an obliteration, of its representation in the brain."[21]

In an attempt to explain the connection between body and self, Sacks muses on the experience of proprioception—"that by which the body knows itself, and has itself as 'property.' One may be said to 'own' or 'possess' one's body—at least its limbs and moveable parts— by virtue of a constant flow of incoming information, arising ceaselessly, throughout life, from the muscles, joints and tendons. One has oneself, one *is* oneself, because the body knows itself, confirms itself, at all times, by this sixth sense."[22] When this flow of information is interrupted through loss of use of a leg or arm, say, a person's ability to know himself or herself through experience of the whole body is compromised.

What does a disease that affects the whole body and is progressive do to one's sense of self? Nancy Mairs considers this question in regard to her MS. When a part of her body doesn't work, she talks about it as an object that exists apart from her. "The left hand doesn't work anymore," for example, or, "There's a blurred spot in the right eye."[23] With progressive MS, however, the damage is so widespread that it cannot be perceived as limited to a particular part, and the effect on the sense of self is particularly devastating. She asks, "Who would I be if I didn't have MS? Literally, no body. I am not 'Nancy +MS,' and no simple subtraction can render me whole. Nor do I contain MS, like a tumor that might be sliced out if only I could find a surgeon brave and deft enough to operate." MS has completely integrated itself into her body: "Physiologically, lesions—sclerotic patches, or plaque, where the nerve sheath has been destroyed and scar tissue has formed in its place—have appeared throughout my brain and spinal cord: they are integrated into my central nervous system just as thoroughly as the remaining healthy tissue."[24]

Mairs wonders whether she would have been left with a more solid sense of self had her disease not been a degenerative one. Would she have accepted what had happened to her and gotten on with her life? Having a degenerative disease and knowing that her situation will worsen, she experiences her self as ever-changing. "How can I believe that my life is real when it feels so desperately provisional? Oddly, I don't consider the lives of other people with disabilities to be similarly inauthentic. Only my own seems flimsy and counterfeit."[25]

Sometimes the experience of disembodiment relates not to a limb but to the mind itself. As the poet and novelist Floyd Skloot describes, chronic fatigue syndrome fundamentally altered his thought processes.[26] When he began writing his memoir he wasn't sure he would be able to write at all. His thought processes were "weirdly disrupted,"[27] he reported, making it impossible to concentrate well or even spell: "words come out all twisted up: *crhnoic* instead of *chronic, does* instead of *dose*)."[28] He attempts to make sense of how his brain, as if independent from him, functions. He concludes that the "Xerox machine apparently stands for all machines in my rearranged brain: I ask my wife to reheat my coffee in the Xerox, ask my son to Xerox the lawn, explain to my daughter that the doctor will Xerox her injured arm."[29] Skloot becomes the instrument through which his brain communicates what is nonsensical to Skloot himself. That he speaks but does not know what will come out of his mouth reflects a fundamental instability of the self. The mind he has always counted on has taken on a life of its own and will act as outrageously as it likes. "What my neuropsychologist has called 'difficulty in keeping track of ongoing mental activity,' I experience as being estranged from my normally reliable mind. Cut off against my will, as though it had walked out on me and left no forwarding address."[30] How then can a person in this situation be asked to function normally?

After many misdiagnoses Laura Hillenbrand, the author of *Sea Biscuit*, was also diagnosed with chronic fatigue syndrome, which she described in an article in the *New Yorker*. Like Skloot, she became aware that her mind was not processing information as it once had. She would look at words or pictures and see only shapes without meaning or at clocks and not know how to interpret the position of the hands. Sometimes she felt that everything was scrambled in her brain. "Words from different parts of a page appeared to be grouped together in bizarre sentences: 'Endangered Condors Charged in Shotgun Killing.' In conversation, I'd think of one word but say something completely unrelated: 'hotel' became 'plankton'; 'cup' came out 'elastic.' I couldn't hang on to a thought long enough to carry it through a sentence."[31] People diagnosed with chronic fatigue syndrome typically experience it as if they are losing their minds. In a sense they must work to think of it as a physiological failure, so as not to be overwhelmed by a sense that the self has been shattered.

The tendency of medicine to focus on disease, as if the body is separate from the person, often contributes to the patient's sense of the body as alien and not quite human. Barbara Ehrenreich describes how, in the course of her diagnosis and treatment for breast cancer, her body was objectified in the medical world. To others she becomes an object, specifically a disease. She quotes her surgeon, who announces, "Unfortunately, there is a cancer,"[32] as if her cancer is an event that bears no relationship to her. This objectification obliterates whatever authority she has in her life. The worst part of hearing her diagnosis is "not the presence of cancer but the absence of me— for I, Barbara, do not enter into it even as a location, a geographical reference point. Where I once was—not a commanding presence perhaps but nonetheless a standard assemblage of flesh and words and gesture—'there is a cancer.'"[33] In addition, she is rendered invisible by technologies designed to track her cancer and measure her physical stamina. "The endless exams, the bone scan to check for metastases, the high-tech heart test to see if I'm strong enough to withstand chemotherapy—all these blur the line between selfhood and thinghood anyway, organic and inorganic, me and it."[34] And the information described in pamphlets about wigs and implants leads her to fear she will become "a composite of the living and the dead."[35] She asks, "And then what will I mean when I use the word 'I'?"[36]

The Disowned Body

Sometimes the sense of alienation from the body reflects an attempt on the part of the psyche to protect the self from an awareness of loss that would threaten its stability. It is as if the psyche cannot tolerate what has happened and therefore shuns, disowns, or repudiates a part of the body. Robert Murphy describes his own emotional detachment from his body and his tendency to refer to one of his limbs as "*the* leg or *the* arm."[37] He sees this tendency as his attempt to "compensate for what otherwise would be an intolerable violation of my personal space."[38] How else would he survive "being lifted, rolled, pushed, pulled, and twisted"?[39] He explains that as his condition has deteriorated, his solution is "a radical dissociation from the body, a kind of etherealization of identity."[40] In recounting her experience while undergoing a bone marrow transplant Christina Middlebrook describes herself in the third person, as a "zoo creature," a designation that connotes an animal or a monster, suggesting she has lost a sense of herself as human. This zoo creature fits exactly a description of her body ravaged by chemotherapy: it has a "puffed face with deadened eyes," and "is very dopey. Its left eyelid sags. Its back is covered by a hideous, pussy rash that itches. The body has no hair, not on its head, its face, arms, legs, underarms, or now-sexless crotch." She also describes the devastation the chemicals wreak inside her body. The zoo creature "cannot swallow. . . . It vomits buckets of blood. . . . Retching, retching, retching."[41]

Middlebrook maintains, however, that the worst part of her experience is that it deprives her of the human functions of thinking, remembering, processing information, writing. "Worst of all, the zoo creature cannot think or remember. It says things in a language that makes no sense. It cannot watch or understand a video, does not read or listen to music."[42] Middlebrook goes on: "Unable to speak but wanting to make contact, it takes a pen in claw and makes scratches over paper in imitation of human writing. . . . The markings wander demented off the page."[43] It is not that the self remains intact as the body suffers the ravages of disease and treatment; the self, deprived of human function, seems less and less human.

For Lucy Grealy it is her face that she attempts to disown. In *Autobiography of a Face* she describes the repeated surgeries performed to repair the damage from removal of part of her jaw because of a childhood bone cancer. They leave her face alternately swollen and bruised, then sunken. Given that a person's face represents most forcefully who he or she is, how is it possible to maintain a positive sense of self in view of damage to that face? Grealy describes the strategies she employed to repudiate, ignore, or avoid her face in order to protect herself from the feelings it would produce in her. She generally refused to look in the mirror or would look but simply not register the face she was actually seeing. Sometimes she would imagine a "real" or "original" face that existed before surgery or tell herself that parts of her character, like her intelligence, were what really mattered.[44]

Significantly, her book ends with Grealy looking at her reflection in a window, an action that suggests she is recognizing the face as her own, accepting that what she sees is actually her face. Knowing now that Grealy committed suicide at the age of thirty-nine, many years after her original diagnosis and some years after the publication of her book, it is difficult not to conclude that in the end she could neither disown nor own her face. She could not accept the damage to her face and her identity. It seems that even her enormous talent and intelligence could not sustain her in view of the continued emotional torment caused by her physical disfigurement. She could not, in the end, hold on to a positive sense of self when the face she presented to the world, her actual face, appeared so damaged.

Sometimes suffering is so severe and so threatens the coherence of the self that the sufferer absents himself or herself emotionally from the experience. In situations of extreme physical or emotional suffering, a psychological withdrawal from the suffering body occurs. In certain instances there is no question of resilience; survival depends on the ability of the self to split off from what is happening. Christina Middlebrook describes a psychic mechanism that protects her from overwhelming pain during her bone marrow transplant. In a chapter called "Witness" she explains that to survive her stem cell transplant, to preserve her self, the self that was being killed off along with her body, she needed to split her self off from her body. "To save myself, *I*, the me of me, retreated to a far corner above the room. From there, I think, I turned my soul away to contemplate the firmament." Because the transplant was so debilitating she, like others who have gone through it, imagined herself somewhere else as a way to protect her "endangered identity."[45]

Middlebrook reports actually remembering the day she removed herself from a sense of connection to her suffering body. Her friend John was visiting. "I took the person he had come to visit and wrapped her in my arms. My body stayed in the bed, robotlike, to push a call button and get to the bathroom. My soul and I departed."[46] This phenomenon, which psychologists call dissociation, is a characteristic response to overwhelming trauma. As Middlebrook says, "Abused children, concentration-camp internees, soldiers under bombardment, all may split off from their bodies."[47] In these cases the experience threatens to overwhelm a person. The pain, the sickness unto death, the compromised ability to think, the sense of suffering that is unending, become simply unbearable.

The necessity of those who suffer to distance themselves either from the alien body part or the overwhelming emotional situation has a parallel in the doctor's situation. Needing both to remain clear-headed and focused on diagnosis and to feel protected from emotional pain, the doctor also creates a distance from the patient's body and experience. Perhaps the author of a triumph narrative also shares this feeling that the experience is too much to bear. In describing the self as resilient, he or she is perhaps pushing away horrifying and unbearable aspects of the experience that would challenge resilience.

Disowned Emotional Suffering

In the case of someone who becomes blind as an adult the very foundation of the self is shaken. This is because a person's sense of self is so intricately bound up with the experience of the body in space and in relationship to other bodies and solid objects. In *Touching the Rock* the professor of religious education John Hull gives us a stunningly perceptive and moving description of his experience as he gradually loses his eyesight until he becomes totally blind in his late forties.[48] Blindness alters every aspect of his experience of self and relationships. Even when he has largely adjusted to his total blindness, Hull can still feel he is losing himself, precisely because it is difficult for him to locate the boundaries of his body; it is as if he is floating in space. And when his awareness of the enormity of his loss of sight threatens to overwhelm him he removes himself either literally or psychically from a situation. This is a more conscious and intentional dissociation than what others like McCrum describe. Hull decides to withdraw to protect himself. For example, sitting in a room with other people, he is struck by the fact that he is unable to make contact with the world beyond his body: he cannot know the room, gaze out, take in the group, speak or make eye contact with someone at a distance. Or he becomes aware of the sounds of activity around him that he cannot identify without sight. When the loss of familiar ways of perceiving begins to undermine his sense of self, he chooses to retreat to his study, where he can feel grounded by the presence of familiar objects like his books, and engage in reading, writing, or another familiar activity.

At other times his retreat is not literal but psychological. The unbearable awareness of what he can no longer do as a father makes him feel drowsy, like being drugged. It is as if something in him shuts down to protect him from a full awareness of all that he has lost: "I hear the children and everyone else whooping with delight, making comments, and it is as if the knowledge which I do have mocks the knowledge which I don't have, while the poignancy of that contrast makes me want to have no more knowledge at all."[49] Hull reports that he is not aware of feeling anger or sadness or self-pity at these times but only the need to withdraw, "as if an intention has taken the place of a feeling. The intention is to withdraw."[50] He becomes interested in the fact that his reaction does not qualify as an emotion, and that his withdrawal actually substitutes for feelings that threaten his stability.

Those who know they are dying but are not in pain may also disown the body and its experience in order to continue to live day to day. In *Stay of Execution* the columnist and author Stewart Alsop describes a "protective mechanism" that keeps him from feeling the full impact of the awareness that he is going to die soon from a rare form of leukemia.[51] He sees this mechanism as partly conscious and reflected in "a decision to allot to the grim future only its share of your thoughts and no more." It is equally part of an unconscious process, much like that experienced by soldiers in war, Alsop suggests: "There is the first sudden shock of realizing that the people on the other side are really trying to kill you."[52] He goes on: "But the incredulity soon wears off, and a kind of unhappy inner stolidity takes over, coupled with a strong protective instinct that the shell or the bullet or the mine will kill somebody else—not me. In this way the unbearable becomes bearable, and one learns to live with death by not thinking about it too much."[53] Alsop's response to his impending death, then, is a kind of denial: death can't really be happening to him and, therefore, he won't think about it too much. As Alsop observes, however, the very psychological mechanism that enables him to bear the unbearable also handicaps him when he comes to describing the terror that overtook him. He notes the "oddly cheerful tone" of much of what he writes when sick.[54]

When, however, a person is actually in the throes of death it becomes impossible to preserve the self. Instead, the self is reduced to, or gives way to, the dying body. When Brodkey refers to the "inability to have an identity in the face of death," he is referring to this dying of the self. He offers a striking description to illustrate what he observed about those near death—they became a dying body devoid of self: "the human form had seemed to pulsate, like a fist opening and closing, moving back and forth from strength to weakness . . . the way the body would open as if into a palm, vulnerable, extended, and then reform into the fist in search of survival. Then, at some point, the fist would not reform itself, and the pulsating would stop."⁵⁵ Here there is no self, only the body gasping out its last breath.

The self as depicted in these narratives is, at least initially, a split self—that is, a self that survives by virtue of its ability to separate itself from or disown diseased parts of the body or aspects of the experience that are too much to bear. People cut off, deny, dissociate from their experience of pain and suffering. This is a depiction of the self far different from that of the triumph narrative in which a unified, resilient self manages illness or disability.

Those who write narratives that recognize the seriousness of damage to the self are engaged in a paradoxical process. On the one hand, they acknowledge the extent to which people survive serious illness or disability by disowning or distancing themselves from the reality of physical devastation that threatens the integrity of the sense of self. On the other hand, by describing the ways they disavow experience they are actually reclaiming those experiences. They attempt to explore in depth the very experience they were trying to escape when ill or injured. They explore the fragility of the self, the severity of the threat to the self, and even the cleverness of the self in finding ways to maneuver around what threatens it. Whereas the writers of the triumph narrative underplay the catastrophe to the self, these untriumphant writers revisit the most devastating aspects of their experience in order to reflect on them. They explore what it is to walk the line between disintegration and survival, and they describe how perilous the journey is. In doing so they reclaim for themselves something of what had been too much to bear. They achieve what Max Lerner calls "the restoration of the selfhood which the dire news had all but shattered."⁵⁶

— CHAPTER III —

Plot: The Disrupted Life

*The body of the cripple was patched and blistered,
and so was the story he would tell.*
—Leonard Kriegel, *Falling into Life*

Most of us have no idea what to say when someone is seriously ill, so we resort to platitudes: "I'm sure you'll be back on your feet in no time" or "Just think about next summer when you will be playing tennis again." Often we tell stories about our friends who also suffered devastating illnesses or injuries but who are now doing just fine, better than expected, in fact, better than ever. These platitudes encapsulate the plot of the triumph narrative—that suffering will result in future recovery and a return to normal life. We have trouble—or resist—imagining a future in which our friend or relative might die or will live with a damaged body, loss of function, and a changed life. Yet this is actually the future for many who are ill. As discussed in the last chapter, those dealing with serious illness or accident find that their internal sense of self is damaged. It is equally true that their sense of self over time is disrupted. In this chapter I will consider the descriptions by writers of how illness or accident changes their sense of who they are as compared to who they were before. Despite assurances from family and friends that they will return to being the person they were before, they often find they do not. They instead must acknowledge the difficulty of accepting and living with a radically changed sense of self.

It is striking to note, when reading illness narratives, how often writers refer to old and new selves as a way to depict how radically the self has been changed. Some mark this radical change by describing in detail the catastrophic event that heralded it—the diagnosis, the accident, or the surgery. Jean-Dominique Bauby, editor-in-chief of the magazine *Elle* in France, wrote *The Diving Bell and the Butterfly* to describe his life after a massive stroke left his body paralyzed except for one eye. He devised a system whereby he would have a person read the alphabet to him and he would blink his eye to indicate the letter he wanted to use. He opens his book with this statement: "No need to wonder very long where I am, or to recall that the life I once knew was snuffed out Friday, the eighth of December, last year."[1] John Diamond in *Because Cowards Get Cancer Too* describes in detail the night before his surgery to remove a cancerous tumor from his tongue. He and his wife have dinner, walk along the Thames, and chat about everything except the operation. He writes, "We drove home and lay together in our bed for what was to be the last time as the couple we had been for eight years. Tomorrow I would become somebody else."[2] Randy Shilts, in *And the Band Played On*, describes the AIDS epidemic as the event that split in two not only individual lives but the life of the gay community. "Before. It was to be the word that would define the permanent demarcation in the lives of millions of Americans, particularly those citizens of the United States who were gay." Shilts goes on: "The epidemic would cleave lives in two. . . . Before meant innocence . . . this was the time before death."[3]

How radical the break between the old and new self is generally reflects the severity and duration of injury or loss of function. Some people initially deny their loss but come to reconcile their experience before and after illness or injury; some try to envision a way to live with multiple experiences of the self, that is, to embrace the new self while also reclaiming or living with the memory of parts of the former self; and finally, some insist the breach between old and new self is absolute and that the sufferer should abandon any hope of returning to his or her previous life. Yet, in fact, even these people retain some connection to who they were in the past. Insofar as the story of illness is the story of the self, this radical change in the self over time becomes a central theme in many narratives and gives rise to an important paradox.

Traditionally autobiographical writing assumes a stable self to be represented in writing through such techniques as chronology, a consistent narrative voice, and plot. Much recent work on autobiography, however, questions the positing of a stable self and suggests instead a more fluid or many-faceted notion of the self.[4] Those who write about their illness and disability are often caught between two characterizations of the self. On the one hand, they want to represent a devastated, broken, or interrupted self, the more complicated self discussed by contemporary theorists of autobiography. On the other, even while proclaiming their old self is gone, they set out to reclaim, in the act of writing, parts of that old self. In this sense they use writing much as traditional writers of autobiography have—to bestow coherence. They talk about their old self, review what has happened to them, and place themselves once again in their own familial or literary ancestry.

Many narratives are characterized, then, by the dual and sometimes conflicting desires of authors both to convey the enormous rift in their lives caused by illness or injury and, through writing, to restore continuity to their experience. These narratives also reflect the difficulty of actually representing a break in the self. However much writers talk about this break in the self over time, they do so in one voice and usually in the context of a chronological story, thereby bestowing a measure of continuity, even more than they may wish to bestow, on the disrupted self they wish to represent.

Denial of Reality

The road to acknowledging this radical change in the self involves a complex negotiation between the need to acknowledge the loss of the old self and then, paradoxically, to reclaim parts of the old self even as a new one develops. Many people initially deal with shifts in self-conception after radical damage to the body through denial. In his narrative *Falling Into Life* Leonard Kriegel describes the various strategies he utilized early on in his polio. As an eleven-year-old, he needed to deny the radical split between his experience of himself before polio—the boy who could walk and run—and the crippled boy he became. Unable to accept his paralysis, he used his "ability to imagine myself whole in body and triumphant in spirit" to protect himself from the harsh reality of his overwhelming loss.[5] In other words, he simply pretended to himself that he could walk and run.

Only later did he accept all that he had lost of the boy he was and to face "the anguish of unfulfilled aspirations."[6]

Kriegel suggests that the move toward a future and creation of an authentic self is always counterpoised with "his growing obsession with the self he was never allowed to possess."[7] He comes to live with his past not by denying what happened to him or by accepting the death of his old self but by letting the possibilities of that old conception of himself, as a boy able to walk and run, exist in his imagination as a parallel experience. He keeps the lost intact self imaginatively alive next to his disabled self. For Kriegel, "It was the disease-ridden imagination that recognized that before the day came that I could claim myself, I would have to claim all my imaginary selves."[8] A person whose body is radically changed inevitably perceives the world differently. When Kriegel left the rehabilitation hospital and returned to his old neighborhood wearing braces and crutches, for example, the neighborhood seemed reconstructed; his slow struggle to cover even a small distance made the neighborhood seem larger. Finally, Kriegel notes, the changes in one's body result in absolute changes in the future. He says, "The ache of talents lost and ambition mocked sealed me within the bitter recognition that disease takes more than the parts of one's body."[9]

Those who have suffered near total paralysis report a radically altered sense of self. Christopher Reeve describes different stages in his movement toward acceptance of his changed body and self. He begins *Still Me* with a description of a movie character he envisions. This character essentially lives in a fantasy, imagining himself whole in body and able to go sailing as he had before he was injured. Reeve, like Kriegel, posits that imagination, with its possibility of envisioning a different reality, functions as a tool for those unable or not yet ready to accept what has happened to them. Reeve's imagined character maintains that, as crazy as it might be to live in a dream, he finds it helps him with his depression. When eventually he is able to accept his situation he gives up his fantasy and lives fully in reality. He is still a quadriplegic in the hospital "But he has an entirely new basis for the future with his family and toward recovery."[10]

For Reeve's character, the fantasy of sailing functioned as a way to bridge the gap between his old and new self. Unable to accept the changed status of his body, he imagines himself as physically whole until he can live authentically in his new life. But Reeve himself explains later in the book that he continued to struggle with the reality of his situation, refusing at times to revisit the memory of his past intact body and self. This is, however, no longer denial so much as a conscious choice; while acknowledging what happened to him he avoids dwelling on it. "I have to stop this cascade of memories, or at least take them out of their drawer only for a moment, have a brief look, and put them back. . . . There is no other way to survive than to be in the moment."[11] Like Kriegel, Reeve disagrees with those who tell him he will adjust and declares instead, "I have found exactly the opposite to be true. The longer you sit in a wheelchair, the more the body breaks down and the harder you have to fight against it."[12]

By naming his book *A Whole New Life* Reynolds Price signals his recognition that his life has been completely changed since a tumor in his spinal column left him confined to a wheelchair. Price is determined not to gloss over reality and insists, paradoxically, that one must accept that the old self is lost before trying to reclaim parts of it. At the end of his book he advises those who have experienced a catastrophic change in their body to accept that they are alone in this experience, that no one can rescue them from it, and that they must face the truth of what has happened. "Your mate, your children, your friends at work—anyone who knew or loved you in your old life— will be hard at work in the fierce endeavor to revive your old self, the self they recall with love and respect."[13] While their intentions may be generous, Price insists their efforts will hinder you in your efforts to come to terms with your changed body. He maintains that the job is to discover, and fast, "that next appropriate incarnation of who you must be, and then *become* that person."[14]

Price's portrayal of people's reassurance as misguided suggests a story of disability that is unsettling, even to those who are critical of the easy assumptions of recovery that characterize the triumph narrative. The best thing anyone could have done for him after he completed his five weeks of radiation treatments, he claims, "would have been to look me square in the eye and say this clearly, 'Reynolds Price is dead. Who will you be now? Who *can* you be and how can you get there, double-time?'"[15] Price goes on: "Your chance of res-

cue from any despair lies, if it lies anywhere, in your eventual decision to abandon the deathwatch by the corpse of your old self and to
search out a new inhabitable body."[16]

Paradoxically, however, while insisting that one abandon one's
old self, Price suggests that a person must manage his or her transformation into a new person "without forgetting the better parts of
who you were."[17] In fact, Price does this in his own memoir. At the
same time that he depicts a radical split in his own life, he keeps
returning in his story to his past. The movement of his story is often
circular: he is brought back and brings the reader back over and over
again to memories of his father and mother, particularly at the time
of their dying. In doing so he places himself back in the predisability
history of his own family and in the chronology of his own life. Price
also goes to great length to recall other writers he has known who
were disabled, thus finding a place among them not only as a writer
but also as a writer who is disabled. He says, "I've tried to map . . . the
ways I traveled toward the reinvention and reassembly of a life that
bears some relations with a now-dead life but is radically altered,
trimmed for a whole new wind and route."[18]

Even when the body can be restored to its former state, or when
the appearance of the formerly intact body can be restored, a person
must still mourn the loss of an earlier conception of self as well as the
loss of a sense of security about life and the future. In regard to breast
cancer the cultural preference for a narrative of triumph as opposed
to a narrative that acknowledges loss is clearly articulated. Breast
reconstruction after a mastectomy is often presented to women not
simply as one of a number of possible choices but as the preferred
choice. Women are told their breasts will be as good as new after
surgery, as if a reconstructed breast will somehow negate the need to
mourn the loss of the original breast. They are often given little sense
of the limits and even drawbacks of that surgery.

Audre Lorde's book *The Cancer Journals*, courageous when first
published, continues to be distinguished from other memoirs about
breast cancer for its insistence that women face their loss, not hide
their changed bodies, and integrate what has happened to them into
their sense of self. In reflecting on her own mastectomy Lorde states,
"Any amputation is a physical and psychic reality that must be inte-

grated into a new sense of self."[19] She believes breast prostheses and reconstruction after cancer interfere with this process.

Yet, she points out, this is not the prevailing belief. She offers examples that illustrate the prevalent, contrary notion—that women can simply return to life as it was before. While in the hospital Lorde is visited by a woman from the organization Reach for Recovery who proudly displays her upright and rigid, implanted breasts. She suggests helpful exercises and encourages Lorde to have a positive attitude. Although Lorde appreciates her practical suggestions and encouragement, she finds her enthusiasm about breast prostheses completely objectionable. "Her message was, you are just as good as you were before because you can look exactly the same. Lambswool now, then a good prosthesis as soon as possible, and nobody'll ever know the difference." Lorde responds, "I knew sure as hell *I'd* know the difference."[20] Lorde believes that a woman whose lost breast is "buried under prosthetic devices . . . must mourn the loss of her breast in secret, as if it were the result of some crime of which she were guilty."[21]

Similarly, ten days after having her breast removed Lorde, feeling good and dressing stylishly, returned to the office of her breast surgeon. The nurse whom she had previously found to be supportive ushered her into the examining room and asked her why she was not wearing a prosthesis. "The nurse now looked at me urgently and disapprovingly as she told me that even if it didn't look exactly right, it was 'better than nothing,' and that as soon as my stitches were out I could be fitted for 'a real form.'"[22] "You will feel so much better with it on," the nurse went on. "And besides, we really like you to wear something, at least when you come in. Otherwise it's bad for the morale of the office."[23] Lorde rejects the notion that these women dealing with breast cancer should have presented themselves as if nothing in their life had changed and suggests that each "could have used a reminder that having one breast did not mean her life was over, nor that she was less a woman, nor that she was condemned to the use of a placebo in order to feel good about herself and the way she looked."[24]

Narratives, of course, hold different meanings at different cultural and historical moments. The notion so central to the triumph narrative, that the body can be made as good as new, was oppressive to Lorde. However, when Betty Rollins published *First You Cry* in 1976, she broke a cultural taboo against speaking about breast cancer. Her narrative of triumph over breast cancer was empowering for women at that time. She maintained that women could survive cancer with a self intact and with self-respect. By demonstrating that life could go on after breast cancer she provided an important alternative to the prevailing notion that breast cancer was shameful, to be hidden and probably a death sentence.

Contemporary women, like Lorde, however, now face a culture that has gone from seeing breast cancer as something shameful to one that expects women to continue on as though nothing has happened, even while they undergo surgery, radiation, and chemotherapy. A woman with breast cancer is praised for continuing to work and care for her family, for having her breasts reconstructed and never talking about the possibility of dying. Improved techniques for breast reconstruction have only lent greater intensity to the widespread insistence that a woman can restore her body to its former state. A woman who learns she has cancer and needs a mastectomy certainly may find this idea appealing: in all this discussion serious consideration of the risks of surgery, the imperfect outcomes, and the not unusual need for repeated surgeries is often underplayed. Perhaps behind this public insistence on the value of reconstruction lies the fear of acknowledging limits and permanent damage and the inability to accept that life does change after cancer.

Multiple Selves

When it comes to mental illness the issue of self can be particularly complicated. Manic depression, for example, is by definition an illness in which the self does not remain constant over time but can change radically from one moment to the next. In many ways manic depression manifests itself in the guise of two selves, hardly compatible in the same person, which seem to alternate with each other at different times rather than exist together in one person. In *An Unquiet Mind* Kay Jamison, a psychiatrist who writes about her own manic depression, describes the identity problems that arise from the discrepancy between the violence of her manic and depressive states and her more normal moods. In her blind, manic rages she is "wildly out of control—physically assaultive, screaming insanely at the top of [her] lungs, running frenetically with no purpose or limit, or impulsively trying to leap from cars."[25] During these attacks, "I . . . destroyed things I cherish, pushed to the utter edge people I love, and survived to think I could never recover from the shame. I have been physically restrained by terrible, brute force; kicked and pushed to the floor; thrown on my stomach with my hands pinned behind my back; and heavily medicated against my will."[26]

Imagine trying to reconcile this kind of violent self with an otherwise well-behaved self. As Jamison describes it: "After each of my violent psychotic episodes, I had to try and reconcile my notion of myself as a reasonably quiet-spoken and highly disciplined person . . . with an enraged, utterly insane, and abusive woman."[27] Sometimes she had to reconcile her normally lively and enthusiastic self with the deadened self of her depression—"a dreary, crabbed, pained woman who desperately wished only for death"[28]—or with the less lively, less creative, more sedate self she feels herself to be when on medication. Like others with manic depression, she must struggle to avoid a return to the very manic state that she actually finds preferable. The liveliness and excitement of that state can easily result in behavior that is out of control and destructive. As a result, Jamison explains, she can never go back, never be that old self without risking further illness, repeated manic episodes followed by serious, perhaps suicidal, depression.

Many of those who are seriously ill and recognize the radical change in self still long for their old self and life and, in fact, attempt as much as possible to reclaim life as it was before. These attempts typically do not so much replace as accompany attempts to accept what has been lost. They signal an acknowledgment of an experience of multiple selves. Many writers describe trying to get back the parts of the former self that have been lost. This involves, first and foremost, taking part again, when possible, in those activities that characterized the old self. For example, McCrum, after his stroke, describes his convalescence as comprising various ways he attempted to reclaim himself through activity. As he put it, "I made a call from a pay phone. I took a train. I flew in an aeroplane. I went swimming. I ordered a meal in a restaurant. I made love to my wife."[29] He lists each of these activities to underscore how significant they were, given that he had not thought he would do them again. "In subsequent months I continued to repossess my experience of the world. I went to the opera *(Don Giovanni)*. I walked alone to post a letter. I got my driving license back. I made—and kept—an appointment to get my hair cut."[30] By resuming the activities of daily life he reconnected with his old self: "Slowly, I recovered pieces of my old way of life, bit by bit, as if reconstructing a scattered jigsaw."[31]

Gaps in the Self

The need to connect present self to past sometimes involves consciously filling in the missing pieces of experience as a way to establish continuity over time and to repair the radical split in the self. Christina Middlebrook explains that she could not remember her experience during her bone marrow transplant, largely because she shut down when it became too much to bear. She didn't "disappear forever during that hideous fight,"[32] she concludes, because those around her, whom she calls witnesses, continued to treat her as the person she had been before. They talked to her, fussed over and cared for her. As she recovered she became determined to reclaim that lost experience. "I want the whole of my life back. I need a continuum from then to now."[33] Middlebrook asked family and friends to recount what happened to her during the transplant. Her husband told her she needed warm blankets; her daughter described her skin; her son recalled the fragile sound of her voice on the phone. Friends described visits and recalled the details of conversations. Middlebrook is able to reclaim only those aspects of the experience for which others were present; otherwise "those events are lost. *I* was not there."[34] So significant is the reclamation of lost experience, however painful, that she suggests it is "the only way the soul survives."[35]

When Gilda Radner was undergoing chemotherapy for ovarian cancer, she devised a playful way to maintain the continuity of her antic self while she was otherwise occupied with chemotherapy. In *It's Always Something* she describes enlisting her husband, Gene

Wilder, to make a video of her playing tennis that would be shown in her room while she slept during chemotherapy. In the video she repeatedly hits the ball, runs and jumps, and makes jokes. Sometimes it is a basketball that comes across the net. Tennis friends applaud her and give testimonials about how well she is playing. She speaks into the camera: "Through the miracle of chemotherapy, I am able to play tennis as badly now as I did before I had cancer."[36] The tape of her hilarious performance plays on for every doctor, nurse, and visitor who enters her room. In this way Radner continues to exist in the minds of others as the comedian they have known her to be. Later on, Wilder also made a videotape for Radner of her entire last chemotherapy treatment. When she watches it, she sees Gene sneaking their dog into the room, the dog kissing Gene, and herself sleeping a lot. The nighttime portion is filmed by the nurse who, to liven up the video, writes notes with supposed quotes from Radner about how happy she is that chemo is over and how well she is doing. Later Radner and the nurse watch it together. Both these filming activities are Radner's way of maintaining the continuity of her self. The tennis video keeps present her self as comedian; the chemo tape her self being treated for cancer.

In a later chapter I will consider how writing itself becomes a way to represent the gaps illness causes in the continuity of life, but here my point is to emphasize how central is the preoccupation with the self that has been lost. Many of the writers I have discussed so far have been able to reclaim much of their former lives. Those who walk on crutches or are confined to a wheelchair can live fairly normal lives. Yet even those who can compensate for lost function stress the need to come to terms with what has been lost and the ways their bodies have been irrevocably changed.

The Radically Altered Self

Often after a serious accident, stroke, or radical surgery, a person emerges feeling like a different person, as if completely cut off from the past, although eventually he or she is able to resume many of the functions temporarily lost. Robert McCrum in *My Year Off* maintains that the person who is damaged by a stroke must mourn the loss of the physically intact body and self and give up hope of returning to that person. McCrum felt so changed that he could barely connect the person he now was to the person he had been before. He reports that his wife feared not only that his mind would be gone or he would be paralyzed but that he would be without joy, a different person entirely. Even when McCrum acknowledges that he functions much like his old self, he insists that at best he is a feebly repaired self. He states that "the cruel fact is that this former self is irretrievably shattered into a thousand pieces, and try as one may to glue those bits together again, the reconstituted version of the old self will never be better than a cracked, imperfect assembly, a constant mockery of one's former, successful individuality."[37]

John Hull writes about his blindness, an experience from which he will not recover. While he does compensate for certain lost functions—he finds a way to read, to walk down the street unaccompanied—there are aspects of his former life that he cannot reclaim: he cannot see the mountains or his children's faces. Hull describes his experience of blindness early on as much like that of an unborn child, a fitting image given that he was embarking on a new life. Having formerly functioned with confidence in the world and having been secure in his movements, he now feels he is going back "into the unborn state, where one is free-floating without distinction, enclosed at the end of a tunnel, without a world and finally without a self."[38]

Hull describes the panic he experiences at the prospect of living in the world without the sense of self he always counted on. Every activity is like venturing out for the first time. In a chapter entitled "Panic in a Mineshaft" he describes leaving his house on a bitterly cold day. After going about a hundred yards, he explains, "I became aware of a growing feeling of doubt. I became intensely aware of the fact that I was walking through nothing." The feeling continued to intensify. "I was alone, entering the night of an endless tunnel of intense cold. I knew that once I went in I would not be able to come back. I would be lost. I had a sense of impending doom."[39] Although he struggled against the fear, it was so severe that he turned back.

In addition to offering powerful descriptions of how terrifying and overwhelming it is to realize the new state of his self, Hull describes the painstaking adjustments he needed to make to avoid succumbing to despair and to find a way to live in this radically altered self. At times his awareness of what he has lost threatens to annihilate him. As time goes on, though, Hull devises ways to fend off panic. In addition to learning Braille and using a seeing eye dog, he devises strategies to avoid the sense that he is lost and without boundaries or self. To keep himself from disintegrating, he needs to feel grounded in a familiar world, he realizes. "Familiarity, predictability, the same objects, the same people, the same routes, the same movement of the hand in order to locate this or that: take these away, and the blind person is transported back into the infantile state where one simply does not know how to handle the world."[40]

To counteract the feeling that he is floating in space, Hull creates boundaries for himself: he makes physical contact with people and things and greets people by taking their hand in both of his. When a task feels overwhelming he breaks it down. For example, rather than think about getting home he thinks about getting to the end of the block. He also sets about restructuring his social interactions. Knowing he needs to participate actively with others, he develops various techniques to compensate for not being able to see who is present in a room with him, make eye contact, or approach people. When it becomes difficult in a social situation to move on from conversation with one person to another he asks the person to whom he is speaking if he or she can introduce him to someone else. As awkward as this is, it keeps him from becoming passive and avoids the danger of losing himself. He makes trade-offs in order to live his new life as a social and independent person. If someone approaches him on the street and offers help he may decline but say he'd enjoy their company. He then takes the person's arm not because he can't walk himself but because walking requires complete concentration and makes it difficult to converse. As he puts it, he gives up his independence for sociability. But then, he explains, it becomes even more complicated. The sighted person comes to think of him as a dependent person, and this alters their relationship.

Hull describes other adjustments he needed to make. He discovers that people often treat him like a child. If he is on the street and asks someone where he is, the person will often reply by asking him where he is going, not understanding that he needs to know where he is in order to orient himself. When Hull wants to sit he finds that people often try to push him into the chair. He therefore asks the person to place his hand on the back of the chair so he can then seat himself.

It is with his own children that Hull feels most in danger of losing himself. He finds himself overwhelmed by a feeling of loss when he is unable to participate at his son's birthday party. He then withdraws to his study where he can ground himself again. Later he sits with his son on the bed and talks with him about each gift the son places in his hands. Gradually Hull builds up a new way to be in relationship to the external world and the people in his life.

Hull shows us how much deeper than a conventional triumph narrative a writer can take us in understanding the actual experience of damage to the body that compromises the self. Without the apparatus of the triumph narrative, he ends up leaving us with a testament to a different kind of triumph—his grappling minute to minute, situation to situation, with how changed his life is from before. He never denies the catastrophe—the loss of sight that resulted in a loss of self—but he takes us through what that loss and adjustment actually entail.

Sometimes the damage caused to a person's body is so extreme and functioning so compromised that a person cannot reconcile his or her past and present self. Those in this situation are no doubt living an entirely different life and are perceived to be a very different person. At the beginning of *Because Cowards Get Cancer Too* John Diamond wonders what happens if he is cured of cancer. "Is that it? Do I go back to being the man I was before?"[41] When Diamond undergoes major surgery to remove the tumor from his tongue, he knows he faces the future as a changed person, perhaps with no tongue and unable to speak. He has no idea who exactly that person will be. "Nobody can tell you how it feels to be that postoperative person, the person who is lying there waiting for the new chapter to start and with no idea of how that chapter will read."[42] What he does expect is that the physical changes will be significant enough to make him feel like a different person. "I knew that everything that had been done to me would have a permanent effect, but I couldn't say what that effect—on my constitution, my looks, my voice, my career, my persona—would be. I lay there and contemplated the new me and was frustrated by the shallowness of contemplation that was possible."[43] He later comes to see, like so many, that the physical damage he incurs from the surgery is accompanied by emotional damage as well.

Diamond discusses an important side effect of the radical change in his physical state: that others may continue to react to him as the person he was or be uninterested in the person he has become. He considers the painful possibility that the people who love him would probably not have been interested in him had they first met him in his present altered state. Always a witty, voluble, and active person, he now struggles to express even the simplest thought and maintain some sense of security. "Would the people I love love me, know me, have taken trouble with me, if this was how I was when they first met me? Would my friends . . . have become my friends if when we first met I'd been a wounded, honking mute unable to respond to the simplest question without dribbling? Would I be with Nigella, come to that? Would I have the kids?"[44]

For Jean-Dominique Bauby, who emerged from a coma in a state called locked-in syndrome, the change in his experience of self was unimaginatively severe. Bauby, like Diamond, describes lying in his hospital bed a changed person. "Paralyzed from head to toe, the patient, his mind intact, is imprisoned inside his own body, unable to speak or move."[45] When he views his twisted and damaged face reflected in the glass he doesn't recognize himself. "Not only was I exiled, paralyzed, mute, half deaf, deprived of all pleasures, and reduced to the existence of a jellyfish, but I was also horrible to behold."[46]

Bauby wonders how one maintains a self at all—old or new—in the face of such devastation. After his stroke he is without the ability to perform most of the bodily functions that comprise the self. And yet he has his mind and imagination. For Bauby there is no question that his old life is gone and he is living a different life. To describe his life he offers the reader the two metaphors of the title. The diving bell—a steel box open only at the bottom, supplied with compressed air through a hose and used by divers descending into the mines— represents his experience in his body. The butterfly—able to fly away—represents his imagination and spirit. The only way Bauby can get through the day and live in any way free of his imprisoned body is to use his imagination to recall the pleasures of places, smells, food, and the people from his past. He also insists on the right to choose his own clothing for the day. Rather than wear the "hideous jogging suit"[47] provided by the hospital, he wears his own clothes. "Like the bath, my old clothes could easily bring back poignant, painful memories. But I see in the clothing a symbol of continuing life. And proof that I still want to be myself. If I must drool, I may as well drool on cashmere."[48] In many ways Bauby is doing what Anatole Broyard suggested in *Intoxicated By My Illness*—developing a style in which to be ill.

Bauby devises an ingenious solution to the problem of communication. After learning that people are describing him as a total vegetable, he decides to mail a monthly letter to his friends as a way of asserting his continued existence as a thinking and communicating person. He develops a painstaking method of "writing" or dictating that involves blinking his one functioning eye. He intends to "prove that my IQ was still higher than a turnip's"[49] and to let the world know that, despite his nearly complete immobility, he is still himself. He receives in response remarkable letters, some serious, some chatty, and imagines making of them "a half-mile streamer, to float in the wind like a banner raised to the glory of friendship."[50] Yet Bauby knows that, even if he keeps the gossips at bay, the grim reality of his paralysis remains unchanged.

Bauby is taken for a ride in his wheelchair by Claude, the woman to whom he is dictating his book, and an old friend, Brice, who tells Claude stories about Bauby's quick temper, his love of books and good food, and his red convertible. Claude comments that she hadn't known he was like that. Bauby realizes, "My present life is divided between those who knew me before and all the others. What kind of person will those who know me now think I was? I do not even have a photo to show them."[51]

For Bauby the split between his old and new self is profound, radical, and unimaginable. He retains only the most limited ability to resume old activities and ways of being in the world—choosing his own clothes and writing this document of his experience. With enormous effort he produces this book that stands as a testament to the continuance of his old self. In a sense he remains the writer and the observer he always was, although he now lives in a paralyzed body and is able to do little but recall his old self. Yet one has the feeling that Bauby keeps a certain distance from his most difficult feelings. Perhaps the book represents a refusal to live only in his present nightmarish situation.

All of these writers who describe serious illness or injury emphasize how radically changed they are from the person they were. Unlike the triumph narrative that suggests a resilient self able to cope with illness or injury, these writers depict a fragile self so altered by illness or accident as to seem a different self. The task of recovering becomes all the more monumental. Those affected must resurrect the old self, or at least the parts of that self they can reclaim; or they must learn to live in a radically changed body and become the person they will be in it. If they do so it is with the painful awareness of all that has changed in themselves over time. While some continuity with the old self of course remains, by referring to the old and new selves these writers suggest how profound is the change in their experience of themselves. They tell a story that focuses, not on external events as they move toward a triumphant end, but on an internal experience of disruption and disorientation.

How, then, does one capture in writing this experience of a self radically altered over time?

CHAPTER IV

Searching for a Language

> *Are words actually any use to describe what pain*
> *(or passion, for that matter) really feels like?*
> —Alphonse Daudet, *In The Land of Pain.*

> *No worse, there is none. Pitched past pitch of grief,*
> *More pangs will, schooled at forepangs, wilder wring.*
> —Gerard Manley Hopkins

How far can anyone go in describing what it is like to be seriously ill or disabled? How can a person represent bodily experience, discomfort, or pain? Or explain suffering, despair, loss, and the fear of dying? I remember my own illnesses, particularly the months of chemotherapy, when I would try to describe the experience—like being sick in every pore, having the flu times a hundred, having Drano in my veins. And yet, none of these descriptions came anywhere near communicating what I was feeling. My sense of isolation was only increased by my frustration at the sheer inadequacy of my attempts to communicate.

Discussion of a language for illness has been largely shaped by Susan Sontag's pathbreaking book *Illness as Metaphor.* Sontag has sensitized us to the judgments inherent in the metaphors used for illness. She concludes, in fact, that it is preferable to avoid using metaphorical language when discussing illness. The writers of many memoirs of illness follow in the tradition of Sontag and offer examples to further demonstrate her point.

There is, however, another discussion about language for illness that is very much alive among writers. Many, in a kind of response to Sontag, are asking the question, "So how then, if we eschew metaphor, do we talk about the physical pain and emotional suffering that we experience when ill or injured?" These writers, while acknowledging Sontag's contribution, go on to consider the value of metaphor in writing about illness. In this chapter I will review Sontag's argument and demonstrate how it informs discussion about a language for illness. I will then consider the critique of Sontag's argument offered by those struggling to describe their experience.

The Problem with Metaphor

In her book Sontag focuses on the implications of numerous metaphors used for TB, cancer, and, in a later edition, AIDS. She argues, for example, that TB, because its cause is unknown, is seen as "an insidious, implacable theft of a life."[1] She points out that when cancer treatment is viewed as analogous to warfare, the necessary treatments become weapons against disease and the ill person becomes a civilian casualty. "There is everything but the body count."[2] She notes that AIDS has come to be viewed as a disease of excess or perversity and has taken on the connotations of a plague—a threat to the community, originating from the outside. So insidious are these metaphors that Sontag suggests we abandon them, "that the most truthful way of regarding illness—and the healthiest way of being ill—is one most purified of, most resistant to, metaphoric thinking."[3]

Perhaps best known is Sontag's discussion of the use of military metaphors for disease. Implicit in the metaphor of battle is a fundamental way of viewing those who are ill: the patient, rather than be viewed as suffering, is expected to fight, struggle, and defeat the enemy that is illness. The greatest tribute, paid in most obituaries to people who die after a long illness, is that they battled bravely. In some sense Sontag's critique of the battle metaphor is essentially a critique of the triumph narrative. Both depict the sufferer as a warrior expected to fight bravely against the evil enemy, the disease.

Many writers explore further the negative implications of the use of this still predominant military metaphor. Nancy Mairs explains that "the afflicted body is never simply that—a creature that suffers, as all creatures suffer from time to time. Rather, it is thought to be . . . 'embattled,' and thus in need of militaristic response, its own or someone else's, to whip it back into shape."[4] John Diamond argues that the "whole battlefield vocabulary suggested that the cure for cancer had a moral basis—that brave and good people defeat cancer and that cowardly and undeserving people allow it to kill them."[5] Barbara Ehrenreich notes that "the words *patient* and *victim*, with their aura of self-pity and passivity,"[6] have been designated politically incorrect, and replaced by active verbs that, unfortunately, are drawn primarily from the military. "Those who are in the midst of their treatments are described as 'battling' or 'fighting,' sometimes intensified with 'bravely' or 'fiercely'—language suggestive of Katharine Hepburn with her face to the wind."[7] These more active words, while most likely intended to empower those who suffer, impose another kind of cultural expectation—that they, in refusing to be victims, become fighters.

Those writers who adopt Sontag's approach often extend her analysis to the language used for their particular disease or disability. Georgina Kleege, for example, argues that the symbolic and negative meanings attached to the word *blind* eventually become attached to the person who is blind. According to Kleege the word *blindness*, as it is used throughout history and today, "connotes a lack of understanding or discernment, a willful disregard or obliviousness, a thing meant to conceal or deceive."[8] She goes on to offer a long list of words used more in their figurative than literal sense: "blind faith, blind devotion, blind luck, blind lust, blind trust, blind chance, blind rage, blind alley, blind curve . . ."[9]

Many metaphors that have become part of our language refer literally to physical stature. These metaphors, Nancy Mairs suggests, often carry judgments about the person whose physical state is represented in the metaphor. Mairs looks at the myriad ways people use metaphor to describe those who, like her, cannot stand. Some attach positive moral qualities to a physical status unavailable to some who are disabled. "'Keep your chin up,' we say (signifying courage), 'and your eyes open' (alertness); 'stand on your own two feet' (independence) 'and tall' (pride); 'look straight in the eye' (honesty)." Others suggest negative moral qualities, for example, "'sit on your ass' (laziness), 'take it lying down' (weakness), 'listen with half an ear' (inattention), and get left 'without a leg to stand on' (unsound argument)."[10]

The Need for Metaphor

While few disagree with Sontag's ideas about the potential pitfalls of metaphorical language for illness, some have argued that such carefulness about language is confining when it comes to describing their actual experience. Their argument stems largely from the fact that they are less interested in how people label them than in describing their own felt experience of illness or disability. Consequently, they wish to have available to them a broad range of possibilities for verbal expression.

In this vein, wishing to find metaphors powerful enough to capture the emotional experience of illness or disability, some writers embrace language that is often dismissed as prejudicial or demeaning. Robert Murphy in *The Body Silent* chooses the word *paralytic* to describe himself. Acknowledging that many people find the term "short and brutally descriptive," he embraces it as an accurate representation of his physical state.[11] Leonard Kriegel suggests that out of concern for political correctness "we have developed a language of prosthetic inkblots" that masks the actual reality of disability and fails to offer access to what disability is really like.[12] Reynolds Price also rejects these terms and prefers "either gimped or crippled—not disadvantaged, specially challenged, or beatified-by-pain."[13] These writers are interested in a language that conveys the reality of physical damage and the intensity of the experience of illness or disability.

Metaphorical language, because a step removed from the actual lived experience, often fails to register accurately the seriousness of a particular illness or injury. Many writers point out that certain metaphors seem too weak for certain experiences, and they propose more effective metaphors. John Diamond notes that a cancerous tumor is referred to as a "bit of a lump."[14] Similarly, *spot* is the euphemism used for Christina Middlebrook's cancer rather than what she calls "the stink words: tumor, metastasis, recurrence."[15] Similarly, the word *depression*, according to William Styron, is "too weak a word for such a devastating illness," and he wonders if "the harsh old-fashioned words: madhouse, asylum, insanity . . . lunatic, madness," come closer to the truth. As Styron puts it, "never let it be doubted that depression, in its extreme form, is madness."[16]

This interest in finding expressive language for describing the personal experience of illness or disability is at the heart of the major critique of Sontag's book. Not surprisingly, some writers who made the decision to write very personally about their own illness or disability fault Sontag for not acknowledging her own breast cancer. They feel that her intellectual approach keeps her and her readers distant from the actual experience of disease or injury. Leonard Kriegel, for example, praises Sontag for changing the ways writers approach illness, but finds that "as perceptive a critic as she is, Sontag is too distant from her own struggle with cancer, too analytical and impersonal, for my taste."[17] Anatole Broyard, while admiring Sontag for her "elegant analyses of how we think about illness and the stigma we attach to it," also finds her analysis too intellectual. He feels Sontag "aims a bit high for the sick man lying flat in his hospital bed" and wonders if perhaps she is throwing "the baby out with the bath" when she suggests a language "most purified of, most resistant to, metaphoric thinking."[18] Robert Lipsyte reports being less measured in his initial response to Sontag.[19] Although he came to appreciate Sontag, he recalls throwing her book across the room when he first read it. At the time his ex-wife was being treated for breast cancer, and Lipsyte felt that Sontag's failure to mention her own cancer played into a cultural tendency to avoid dealing with cancer.

In Sontag's defense, it is not clear that she ever expected her critique of metaphor to be taken quite so literally. When, in 1989 she added the section on AIDS to her book *Illness as Metaphor*, she responded to her critics by saying, "Of course, one cannot think without metaphors."[20] She explains that when she wrote *Illness as Metaphor* she made a decision not to add her personal story of cancer to the many already written but instead to pursue an idea "to calm the imagination" by demonstrating "that the metaphoric trappings that deform the experience of having cancer have very real consequences."[21] Given that Sontag has successfully demonstrated this, other writers are now pursuing the question of what language can be used effectively to describe personal experiences of illness and injury.

Employing Metaphor

In the opening of her book *The Camera My Mother Gave Me* Susanna Kaysen manages to embody in language her frustration as she tries to describe the pain she feels in her vagina. This passage, while humorous, is actually quite illustrative of the inherent difficulty in describing pain. She moves back and forth between direct description and metaphor, finding one and then the other inadequate. She leads us to understand that she simply cannot find a vocabulary sufficiently nuanced and descriptive for the body and pain.[22]

Kaysen points out that women do not generally know how a vagina, spleen, or a pancreas feels because these parts of their body are generally without sensation. The fact that she feels her vagina means that "it is either erotically engaged or ill." Finding little direct language to describe her irritated and pained vagina, she resorts to metaphor. "Some days my vagina felt as if somebody had put a cheese grater in it and scraped. Some days it felt as if someone had poured ammonia inside it. Some days it felt as if a little dentist was drilling a little hole in it."[23] She tries to explain her pain to her boyfriend. "There's a firecracker in there, I said. It's like a sore throat—I thought this was a helpful image. It's similar to a throat anyhow, so this is a really sore throat. So sore you don't want to swallow, you know that kind of sore throat?"[24] Although she finds enough promise in the metaphor of the sore throat to keep using it, her frustration is evident as she attempts to wrest meaning from the comparison. First she says it's like a sore throat; then a really sore throat; then like a throat so sore you cannot swallow. We feel the ground slipping from under her as she discovers that metaphors seem as feeble as direct language when it comes to describing bodily sensation and pain.

This passage from Kaysen is illustrative of the situation many find themselves in when describing bodily experience. They try everything and yet are still frustrated by the inadequacy of their description. Anatole Broyard offers, in contrast to Sontag's cautionary treatise on metaphorical language, a kind of artistic manifesto for the possibilities of metaphor. He urges the sick person to develop a style in which to be ill and suggests that language and metaphor can be a way to express outrage, impudence, or humor. Broyard uses quite extravagant metaphors that express the persona he has adopted in view of his prostate cancer. Often his metaphors are sexual and suggest his desire to be seen as sexual even in the face of devastating cancer. He compares his cancer to "a love affair with a demented woman who demanded things I had never done before."[25] Elsewhere he says, "My libido is lodged not only in my prostate, but in my imagination, my memory, my conception of myself, my appreciation of women and of life itself. . . . When the cancer threatened my sexuality, my mind became immediately erect."[26] He muses, "As I understand it, the prostate gland is like a raging bull in the body, snorting and spreading the disease." He views his various treatments as designed to tame the prostate. "There's room for hermeneutics here. Is desire itself carcinogenic?"[27]

Equally central to Broyard's identity is his artistic sense; he wants his doctor to be a poet. "The technicians bring in the raw material. The doctor puts them into a poem of diagnosis. So I want a doctor with a sensibility. . . . Imagine having Chehkov, who was a doctor, for your doctor."[28] He also wants his doctor to "be able to imagine the aloneness of the critically ill, a solitude as haunting as a Chirico painting. I want him to be my Virgil, leading me through my purgatory or inferno, pointing out the sights as we go."[29] These images and Broyard's own voice celebrate all he loves in his life—women, poetry, art—and represent a kind of triumph of libido, sexuality, and creativity over illness and dying.

As eloquent and at times thrilling as Broyard's writing is here, his intention is to depict himself as the sexual and artistic man he has been, not as a man who is dying. While he rehabilitates metaphor to describe his illness, he uses it his way, not as an entrance into but as a distraction from his experience in a dying body, as a refusal to die before he does. Excited by his illness, grateful for the literary inspiration it offers him, he writes a variation on the triumph narrative, although certainly not a clichéd one. Yet he does something different in his essay about his father's death from prostate cancer. There, metaphor becomes his way to move deeply into the pain of the experience. Arriving at his dying father's hospital room, he registers his own disbelief: "But my father wasn't in there. Sprawled on a table, incredibly out of place, lay a plastic Prometheus, middle-aged and decrepid, recently emptied by an eagle, varnished and highly glazed as though still wet."[30] He goes on, "Or perhaps . . . an eviscerated old rooster, plucked white, his skin shiny with a sweat more painful than blood. . . . Whatever it was, it wasn't my father."[31] In this instance Broyard proves metaphor a powerful tool for representing the suffering physical body.

The writers I discuss here, in their struggle to describe their experience, try everything they can—direct language, metaphor, simile, allusion—to shed light on those aspects of illness that so often remain in shadow. The task they set themselves is to find a language that can represent the felt experience, particularly those aspects of illness that are underrepresented in the triumph narrative. They struggle to describe physical pain, emotional suffering, the way bodily damage affects the self, and, especially, these aspects of illness that seem indescribable, like grief, despair, and terror.

Language for Physical Pain

Alphonse Daudet, the nineteenth-century French novelist and essayist, kept notes about the chronic physical pain he experienced as a result of the syphilis he lived with for many years. He struggled to find ways to describe both his chronic pain and his emotional suffering, yet he often felt that his efforts were unsuccessful. For example, he says, "How much I suffered last night, in my heel and in my ribs. Sheer torture . . . there are no words to express it, only howls of pain could do so." Or, as he continues, "Words only come when everything is over, when things have calmed down. They refer only to memory, and are either powerless or untruthful."[32] Caught between the impossibility of describing pain and the need to do so, Daudet continues to try. He speaks both directly and in metaphor to describe the actual, physical pain in his body: "Strange aches; great flames of pain furrowing my body, cutting it to pieces, lighting it up." In another passage, "A burning feeling in the eyes. The hideous pain from light reflected in a window."[33] Or later, "Sometimes, on the sole of the foot, an incision, a thin one, hair-thin. Or a penknife stabbing away beneath the big toenail."[34]

At other times he tries to describe the terror he feels when physical symptoms overtake him. "Crossing the road: terrifying. Eyes don't work anymore, can't run, often can't even hurry."[35] He writes short, incomplete sentences to communicate the starkness of his pain, as if there is little to say or because pain prevents him from saying more. Twice, when trying to write while in the throes of terrible pain, Daudet comments on the inadequacy of his own writing. The first time he is trying to describe a particular pain and where it is located in his body. "Morphine injection. Several times in a certain part of my leg. Result: a stinging followed by an unbearable burning feeling in the back, the upper torso, the face and the hands. A subcutaneous feeling, doubtless insignificant but still terrifying: you feel you're heading for an apoplectic fit." He then comments, "The above written during one of these crises."[36] This comment highlights the fact that Daudet is aware—and perhaps reflecting on—the ineffectiveness of his description even when it is written while in pain.

In another passage Daudet comments on the inadequacy of his description of the emotional experience of illness: "Sterility. That's the only word that gets close to describing the horrible stagnation into which the mind can fall. It's the condition believers call accidie." He then comments, significantly, on his own description: "This note, made quickly, is wooden, inexpressive, solipsistic; but it was written during cruel illness."[37] Here Daudet himself suggests that the inadequacy of his description is due to the fact that he is in excruciating pain. Perhaps writing at all was an achievement.

The metaphors Daudet chooses describe his actual bodily experience more successfully than does direct language. For example, Daudet describes how he must concentrate on walking straight: "Fear of an attack: shooting pains that either nail me to the spot, or twist me around so that my foot pumps up and down like a knife-grinder's."[38] This often remarked upon image, by suggesting the movement of his pained body, suggests how completely physical pain contorts his body. In another place Daudet compares himself to Don Quixote, not to make a point about his lordliness or delusions of lordliness, but to indicate the excruciating nature of his pain. "I'm a poor old wounded Don Quixote, sitting on his arse in his armour at the foot of a tree. Armour is exactly what it feels like, a hoop of steel cruelly crushing my lower back. Hot coals, stabs of pain as sharp as needles."[39]

Elaine Scarry explores the question of why physical pain so eludes description. She attributes the profound gulf that exists between the person who is suffering and other people as due not only to the self-absorption caused by pain but to something in the nature of pain itself, namely, that one person's pain cannot be seen by the other; it is simply not available to any of the other's senses. "When one hears about another person's physical pain, the events happening within the interior of that person's body may seem to have the remote character of some deep subterranean fact, belonging to an invisible geography that, however portentous, has no reality because it has not yet manifested itself on the visible surface of the earth."[40] While people feel love or hate for someone or hunger for something, physical pain is without an object; it is for no one or no thing. Scarry argues that it "is precisely because it takes no object that it, more than any other phenomenon, resists objectification in language."[41]

Scarry focuses her discussion on the effort of the person suffering pain to move, through language, to communication of that experience. She quotes Virginia Woolf, who in her essay "On Being Ill" bemoans the fact that the English language "which can express the thoughts of Hamlet and the tragedy of Lear has no words for the shiver or the headache"[42] and who comments that the "merest schoolgirl when she falls in love has Shakespeare or Keats to speak her mind for her, but let a sufferer try to describe a pain in his head to a doctor and language at once runs dry."[43] But these problems are not unique to the English language, Scarry points out. Even Greek, the language of tragedy, while at times more expressive than English, falls short when it comes to representing the most complex and even unnamable emotions. She notes, for example, that Sophocles' description of Philoctetes uttering "a cascade of *changing* cries and shrieks that in the original Greek are accommodated by an array of formal words (some of them twelve syllables long), but that at least one translator found could only be rendered in English by the uniform syllable 'Ah' followed by variations in punctuation (Ah!

Ah!!!!).”[44] The human expression of pain or suffering often resides in the utterances of a wordless sound or a word whose sound is its significance.

Many writers refer to the stark sound of someone in grief or pain. Paul Monette, in his memoir about the death of his lover, Roger, from AIDS, describes how Roger, when he learned he was blind, could only utter a “frail and broken ‘Oh.’” Monette helped Roger telephone people so he could tell them of his terrible loss. Eventually Roger “let the cry tear loose. ‘I’m blind,’ he wailed as he clutched the phone, again and again, to everyone we called.”[45] Monette goes on to say that none of the feeble consolation people tried to offer “will ever mute a decibel of that wail of loss.”[46] Reynolds Price, in a discussion of how people bear agonizing pain, quotes Shakespeare’s *King Lear*: “The worst is not / So long as we can say ‘This is the worst.’” To this Price adds his own thought: “At the actual worst, presumably, we’ll be mute as rocks. Or howling, wordless, or humming nonsensical hymns to any conceivable helper.”[47] The wordless quality of terrible pain presents serious problems for the writer. While Monette can refer to Roger’s heart-wrenching wail of loss, is there really any way to translate that sound to the page? At best a writer can refer to the sound, as Monette does.

Language for Emotional Suffering

The biographer of Virginia Woolf, Hermione Lee, closely examines Woolf’s own attempts to describe her emotional suffering when in the throes of a depressive episode. Having argued that most of the descriptions of Woolf’s suffering offered by others tend to focus on her behavior rather than her own experience, she turns to Woolf’s own descriptions. Lee cites passages that comprise a record of Woolf’s painstaking and tortured efforts to put her pain into words. These entries were written not while Woolf was ill—she couldn’t write then—but later on. They demonstrate how frustrating and even futile Woolf found the task of finding words for her pain.

In these passages Woolf struggles to find language to describe her physical and emotional anguish. For example, Lee quotes Woolf as saying, “I know the feeling now, when I can’t spin a sentence, and sit mumbling and turning; and nothing flits by my brain which is as a blank window. So I . . . go to bed . . . such an exaggerated tiredness; such anguishes and despairs; and heavenly relief and rest; and then misery again. Never was anyone so tossed up and down by the body as I am, I think."[48] Woolf includes a passage called "A State of Mind" in which she again tries to describe her experience. "Woke up perhaps at 3. Oh its beginning its coming—the horror—physically like a painful wave above the heart—tossing me up. I'm unhappy unhappy! Down—God, I wish I were dead. Pause. But why am I feeling this? . . . Wave crashes. I wish I were dead! I've only a few years to live I hope. I can't face this horror any more."[49] Woolf then comments: "This goes on; several times, with varieties of horror."[50] In doing so she seems to remove herself from the attempt to describe her suffering, as if it is futile to try to describe the experience further. Woolf uses direct language—"misery," "horror," "anguishes," "despairs"— in an attempt to capture the overwhelming impact of her depression. Woolf's use of short phrases and dashes for punctuation underline the panic and dread she experiences in the throes of a depressive episode. This passage does not flow but rather has a choppy quality that suggests Woolf's turmoil. The image of a wave rushing to overtake her recurs. Yet Woolf finds that even these carefully considered attempts fail to capture the real feeling of depression. Her comment that "this goes on and on several times, with varieties of horror" suggests that Woolf can go no further in her descriptions.

In another entry quoted by Lee, Woolf offers this description: "I wish I could write out my sensations at this moment. . . . A physical feeling as if I were drumming slightly in the veins: very cold: impotent: and terrified. As if I were exposed on a high ledge in full light. Very lonely . . . Very useless. No atmosphere round me. No words. Very apprehensive. As if something cold and horrible—a roar of laughter at my expense were about to happen. And I am powerless to ward it off: I have no protection. And this anxiety and nothingness surround me with a vacuum." Woolf then makes an odd comment about her thighs in an attempt to locate her suffering. "It affects the thighs chiefly . . . the exposed moments are terrifying. I looked at my eyes in the glass once and saw them positively terrified."[51] Woolf acknowledges the difficulty of describing her illness—"No words," but still she tries to find words to describe the feeling—"cold," "impotent," "terrified," "apprehensive." Yet these words and her reference to her thoughts do little to inform us of the severity of her fear.

In her essay "On Being Ill" Woolf reflects on the question of language for illness. While not as raw as the writing in her diary, Woolf's observations in the essay reflect her intimate knowledge of the limits of language; she explains that the person who is ill "is forced to coin words himself, and, taking his pain in one hand, and a lump of pure sound in the other . . . so to crush them together that a brand new word in the end drops out."[52] Woolf is suggesting not imagistic language but words whose significance lies in their sound. A cry, a wail, or a scream of pain—all expressions of the deepest kind of anguish, are sounds, not words or images.

Connection between Body and Self

Because simile, metaphor, and analogy suggest both literal and figurative meanings at once, some writers use them as a way to depict the interplay of the experience of the body and of the self in illness and disability. Nancy Mairs uses the term *waist-high* throughout her book in both its literal and metaphorical sense: *Waist-high* describes her actual physical state and her angle of vision—what she literally sees from her position in her wheelchair; it is also a metaphor for the fact that she, as a crippled woman, sees the world from a different perspective. "I ask you to read this book, then, not to be uplifted, but to be lowered and steadied into what may be unfamiliar, but is not inhospitable, space. Sink down beside me, take my hand, and together we'll watch the waists of the world drift past."[53] When she says "not to be uplifted," she suggests as well that she is not writing an inspirational, "uplifting" story about triumph over disability but a down-to-earth story about how she makes her life in a wheelchair livable. Hers is a physical as well as a metaphorical position. As always she is reminding us that "Disability is at once a metaphorical and a material state."[54] Her angle of vision, although literally restricted, in fact allows her a different and rich perspective on the world.

A similar attention to both literal and figurative meaning characterizes Kriegel's use of the phrase "falling into life" throughout his book.[55] In order to avoid injury as a child with polio, Kriegel had to learn not to resist but join in the falls that would inevitably occur when he walked on crutches. Figuratively, he needed to learn to fall into life, to accept his paralysis and give himself over to his changed situation. Later in the book Kriegel offers another example of the "falling into life" required of him as an adult. After having dinner in a restaurant with friends he steps out into the rainy night and slips and falls on the street. This time he is unable to get up and needs help from his friends. He observes that, as a middle-aged man, he must accept the literal fact of his physical inability to get up by himself; metaphorically he needs to accept his vulnerability and depend on people. Kriegel anticipates the final lesson will be falling into death, that is, accepting that ultimately his body will fail him completely.

By entitling his book *A Leg to Stand On* Oliver Sacks uses the phrase literally to describe his physical situation—because he broke his leg while hiking on a mountain in Norway, he no longer had a leg to stand on. But the phrase is equally descriptive of his emotional situation—his doctors give no credence to what he is saying about his body. As discussed in chapter 1, Sacks is unable to convince his doctors that he has no sensation in his leg.[56] Because to their eyes his leg appears physically sound, they consider his point of view without foundation; consequently, he has no leg to stand on. Sacks's metaphor is powerful precisely because it describes the literal reality of his physical state and serves as a metaphor to represent his position vis-à-vis his doctors. Each of these authors chooses a metaphor that points to an actual physical situation and then moves from there to suggest something about their experience living in their body.

Indescribable Suffering

There are aspects of physical and emotional pain that are repeatedly referred to by writers as indescribable, elusive, unbearable, or unknowable. These words are generally employed to suggest emotions that lie outside ordinary experience, at the extreme end on a continuum of suffering—despair, unbearable loss, fear of death. The repeated use of these words in place of a more expressive description of a particular experience highlights the problem: there is something about these experiences that cannot be controlled by language and that defies expression.

Those writing about depression most often refer to the indescribability of their experience. Yet their discussion is relevant to many aspects of serious illness. For one thing, depression is a common reaction to the pain, loss of control, and awareness of mortality that characterize catastrophic illness or injury. Writing in the *New York Times* after Spalding Gray committed suicide, Verlyn Klinkenborg refers to Gray's depression, the experience without words, that found expression in the form of a monologue: "It allowed him to weave the story around the story he found impossible to tell, the one without language that led him to take his own life."[57] William Styron alludes throughout his memoir to the slippery nature of depression, suggesting that "depression is a disorder of mood, so mysteriously painful and elusive in the way it becomes known to the self—to the mediating intellect—as to verge close to being beyond description. It thus remains nearly incomprehensible to those who have not experienced it in its extreme mode."[58] In fact, Styron's purpose in writing *Darkness Visible* has to do with the indescribability of the experience; aware that people suffering from depression bear the additional burden of feeling others cannot understand, he tries to enlighten those who have not been depressed about the nature of depression.

Styron's writing about depression bears similarities to Virginia Woolf's, particularly in the way Styron alternates between attempts at description and then dissatisfaction with those descriptions. Sometimes his descriptions are not particularly evocative. He attributes to his depression "a sense of self-hatred . . . a failure of self-esteem."[59] He calls his depression his "dank joylessness"[60] and explains that he was "nearly immobilized and in a trance of supreme discomfort."[61] Perhaps because these descriptions are not particularly evocative, he tries again. He describes "panic and dislocation, and a sense that my thought processes were being engulfed by a toxic and unnameable tide that obliterated any enjoyable response to the living world."[62] People who are healthy, he suggests, cannot "imagine a form of torment so alien to everyday experience."[63] Sometimes he declares his own attempts at description inadequate. "For myself, the pain is most closely connected to drowning or suffocation—but even these images are off the mark."[64] The great American psychologist William James struggled with depression for years and, according to Styron, finally gave up his "search for an adequate portrayal, implying its near-impossibility." He quotes James: "It is a positive and active anguish, a sort of psychical neuralgia wholly unknown to normal life."[65]

Andrew Solomon's *The Noonday Demon* is an eloquent and masterful exploration of the manifestations, history, and treatments of depression as well as a description of his own harrowing personal experience. Solomon, acknowledging what he calls the "linguistic vagary attached to emotional vagary" that characterizes descriptions of depression,[66] goes further than other contemporary writers in finding a descriptive language for depression. His matter-of-fact accounts are powerfully evocative, as when he describes his depression as emotional collapse that manifests itself as physical collapse. "Such depression takes up bodily occupancy in the eyelids and in the muscles that keep the spine erect. It hurts your heart and lungs, making the contraction of involuntary muscles harder than it needs to be.[67] Solomon describes quite brilliantly the experience of what he calls losing his mind, feeling the collapse of logic. He was listening to the conversation at a dinner party. "Someone had said something about China, but I wasn't sure what. I thought someone else had mentioned ivory, but I didn't know whether it was the same person who'd been talking about China, though I did remember that the Chinese had made ivory things. Someone was asking me something about a fish, perhaps my fish? Whether I'd ordered fish? Whether I liked fishing? Was there something about Chinese fish?"[68] At this point his dinner companions recognized something was very wrong and took him home. Solomon realized that by not telling them about his depression and the medication he was on he left them to speculate about other possibilities like drugs, alcohol, or physical disease.

Although this direct description itself is quite powerful, Solomon believes that depression "can be described only in metaphor and allegory."[69] He explains that mild depression "undermines people the way rust weakens iron."[70] He goes on: "If one imagines a soul of iron that weathers with grief and rusts with mild depression, then major depression is the startling collapse of a whole structure.[71] Elsewhere he uses the analogy of a vine choking a tree: "It was hard to say where the tree left off and the vine began. The vine had twisted itself so entirely around the scaffolding of tree branches that its leaves seemed from a distance to be the leaves of the tree." And again, "My depression had grown on me as that vine had conquered the oak; it had been a sucking thing that had wrapped itself around me, ugly and more alive than I. It had had a life of its own that bit by bit asphyxiated all of my life out of me."[72]

In the face of what feels indescribable in their experience, many authors draw on the writings of others. Styron points out that "since antiquity—in the tortured lament of Job, in the choruses of Sophocles and Aeschylus—chroniclers of the human spirit have been wrestling with a vocabulary that might give proper expression to the desolation of melancholia."[73] In this vein, he mentions Shakespeare, Emily Dickinson, Gerard Manley Hopkins, John Donne, Hawthorne, Dostoyevsky, Poe, Camus, Conrad, and Virginia Woolf.[74]

It is striking to note how many writers resort to quoting the same few biblical or literary passages to describe their most extreme suffering—particularly the story of Job, Dante's *Divine Comedy*, and passages from the metaphysical poets describing the "dark night of the soul." These texts, because they so aptly represent the experience of emotional suffering that threatens to annihilate the self, become a kind of shorthand, a metaphorical vocabulary whose meaning is assumed to be all but universally understood. And yet the language of these passages is surprisingly devoid of evocative images; instead it connotes absence, nothingness, darkness, and confusion. It is a language that suggests the kind of anguish that is dark and turned in on itself.

What is it about the story of Job that causes so many to invoke it? Styron himself opens his book with a quote from Job:

> For the thing which
> I greatly feared is come upon me,
> and that which I was afraid of
> Is come unto me.
> I was not in safety, neither

had I rest, neither was I quiet;
yet trouble came.[75]

These lines suggest the feeling that trouble arrives for no reason, that one's worst fears are being realized. They suggest how random is the arrival of disruption in the middle of one's life. Job, a good man, finds no explanation for his suffering; it cannot be explained as punishment. Like many who are ill, Job expects his suffering will end—only to discover more adversity awaits him. In his struggle to resist despair, even as his troubles mount, and to hold on to something meaningful, Job embodies the kind of profound, anguished suffering many who are ill feel.

But for many people, as Styron points out, it is Dante who best captures the experience so often characteristic of serious illness or accident: "In the middle of the journey of our life / I found myself in a dark wood, / For I had lost the right path."[76] The experience of finding oneself in what Dante calls "this fathomless ordeal"[77] and what Styron calls "the unknowable, the black struggle to come" is similar to that of Job.[78] Dante's metaphor, like the passage from Job, captures the shock of having one's life halted abruptly, of finding oneself in the middle of a frightening experience, and of having no way to understand what is happening. The repeated invocation of these lines suggests there is something comforting about the way they capture this experience and about the fact that others have felt equally as bereft. At the same time one wonders if this repeated reference to Dante suggests that even our best writers throw up their hands in frustration when it comes to describing their darkest experiences.

In *A Leg to Stand On* Oliver Sacks quotes Job, Dante, and the metaphysical poet John Donne. Unlike Styron, who focuses on the unexpected arrival of trouble for Job, Job's experience of chaos and the possibility of death resonates with Sacks. He reports that he had been experiencing, especially at night, "frightful, empty images of nothingness" as the result of his terrified, anguished reaction to the lack of movement in his leg.[79] In addition, the failure of his doctors to comprehend what he is saying about the loss of sensation leaves him feeling completely lost and destabilized. "Now, doubly, I had no leg to stand on; unsupported, doubly, I entered nothingness and limbo."[80] This is Sacks's "dark night of the soul."[81] He felt he had lost all "the cognitive and intellectual and imaginative powers" that had aided him in the past, that he "had fallen off the map, the world, of the knowable."[82] Sacks found the metaphysical poets offered not only a depiction of the dark night of the soul but also a kind of resurrection story.

A corollary to the way writers reference these passages is their repeated use of two metaphors for illness—night and another country—which often appear in the titles of the books.[83] Interestingly, Dante's image of a "dark wood" suggests both these dimensions of experience: darkness suggesting something unknown and feared and wood suggesting a different and unfamiliar place. Sontag, despite her admonition to avoid metaphor for describing illness, opens her own book with these two most often invoked metaphors: "Illness is the night-side of life, a more onerous citizenship. Everyone who is born holds dual citizenship, in the kingdom of the well and in the kingdom of the sick. Although we all prefer to use only the good passport, sooner or later each of us is obliged, at least for a spell, to identify ourselves as citizens of that other place."[84]

In some sense the most effective language for capturing those aspects of suffering that feel indescribable may be that which is more connotative than imagistic, that is, language that suggests and evokes a particular feeling. For this reason poetry may contain rich possibilities for representing what is difficult to describe. Certainly the effectiveness of the poetry of Gerard Manley Hopkins is due in large part to the powerful feelings that are evoked by the sound of the words he chooses. The alliteration in a line like "Pitched past pitch of grief," with its hard and repetitive consonant sounds, evokes a sense of heaviness, darkness, despair.[85]

If language proves inadequate for describing extreme anguish, perhaps other forms of artistic expression or representation hold more promise. Styron considers this possibility in regard to depression. He discusses the scene in Bergman's early film *Through a Glass Darkly* when the young woman in the throes of a psychotic depression hopes for a sign from God but instead sees "a monstrous spider that is attempting to violate her sexually."[86] As horrific as this image is, Styron feels it falls "short of a true rendition of the drowned mind's appalling phantasmagoria."[87] Interestingly, Elaine Scarry also considers Bergman's attempts to represent pain. She notes that Bergman in *Cries and Whispers* uses two hundred shades of background red in "a sustained attempt to lift the interior facts of bodily sentience out of the inarticulate pre-language of 'cries and whispers' into the realm of shared objectification."[88] But she feels that ultimately his effort falls short.

Film, like drama, also offers the possibility of suggesting interior states through the movements and nonverbal cues of the actor. In an interview in the *New York Times* Michael Cunningham discusses the ability of the actors in his movie *The Hours* to communicate the depression or anguish of the characters they portray through the slightest movement of their bodies. He notes Meryl Streep's "ability to separate an egg with a furious precision that communicates more about Clarissa's history and present state of mind than several pages of prose might do."[89] He describes another moment later: "And when she finally begins to lose her desperate composure there's a moment—a half-moment, you miss it if you blink—when she literally loses her balance, tips over to the left, and immediately rights herself. If there's a way to do things like that on paper, I haven't found it." [90] He notes a similar kind of physical expressiveness in Juilanne Moore's "face when she looks at her son with an agonizing mix of adoration and terror, knowing she will harm him no matter what she does."[91]

Styron, in his search for a way to represent depression, considers the possibility that artistic renderings other than writing may more successfully represent depression. "In many of Albrecht Dürer's engravings there are harrowing depictions of his own melancholia; the manic wheeling stars of Van Gogh are the precursors of the artist's plunge into dementia and the extinction of self."[92] Musical representations, Styron believes, can evoke something of the feeling of depression. "It is a suffering that often tinges the music of Beethoven, of Schumann and Mahler, and permeates the darker cantatas of Bach."[93] In the end, however, Styron feels that even these attempts by the greatest artists fail to represent adequately the torment of depression.

What I wish to emphasize here is that the best writers, discouraged with their own attempt to represent suffering, try everything they can to find a more adequate way to describe these experiences. They try direct language. They try metaphor. They quote other famous writers. Finally, they consider the possibilities of films, painting, or music for depicting the emotional pain. Their frustrated search itself informs us about the extent to which illness and injury feel unmanageable and beyond language.

The Dying Self

The experience of dying involves the ultimate confrontation with the limits of language. Feeling overwhelmed and anguished at the prospect of dying, those who are ill or injured rely on the same literary tactics as those trying to describe suffering. In his book *Wrestling with the Angel* the journalist Max Lerner describes his heart attack, two cancers, and his approach to his death in his eighties. Like other writers, he chooses passages that refer to darkness and another country. He quotes the biblical passage about Jacob wrestling with the angel to describe his own struggle "with the unfathomable mysteries, with Jacob's angel, with the dark man who came in the night and stayed and left."[94] He also quotes a variety of writers. Thomas Wolfe wrote: "I've made a long journey and been to a strange country, and I've seen the dark man very close."[95] Robert Frost's poetry resonates with him ("I have been one acquainted with the night")[96] as do the words of C. G. Jung, "We do not become enlightened by imagining figures of light but by making the darkness conscious."[97] Finally Lerner quotes the novelist F. Scott Fitzgerald: "In the dark night of the soul it is always three o'clock in the morning."[98] To this Lerner adds his own thoughts about facing death: "I wrestled with this specter, as I did with others, in the lonely watches of the night."[99]

In employing the image of night Lerner, like many writers, is evoking something elemental, unknown, frightening, and yet formless, without boundaries or detail. These references to night, however vague, have an almost universal meaning and suggest an experience generally understood but difficult to describe. Lerner, like many, refers to night in both its literal and figurative sense. Night is actually the time when the fear of death takes over. And night is, metaphorically, the time when a person encounters his or her darker feelings. Lerner describes conversing with a colleague who was growing "eloquent about achieving a society purged of all its traumas and injustices." Facing his own imminent death, Lerner reacted strongly to this notion that life can be purged of pain. He offered his friend, as he does the reader, a kind of manifesto for darkness. "Don't take my night away," he told his friend. "For it is in the night of our being that we fulfill our nonrational needs, from honor to love to belief, and tangle with the sometimes tragic, sometimes absurd, fiber of our lives."[100]

Elsewhere Lerner describes in terms of darkness the kind of vulnerability and regression a man in his eighties feels as he approaches death. His wife is out and he has finished dinner with his adult son and son's friend who are on their way to a movie. He asks them to stay with him and they do, but he then wonders what he was afraid of. "Obviously death that might come not as some grand climax but in the midst of life's routines." At the age of eighty he finds himself asking his grown son to stay home with him, "as a child at bedtime begs his parents not to leave him in the dark."[101] "I was afraid of the 'dark.' More nakedly and simply, I was afraid to die."[102]

When death is expected but physical pain not severe, people can think and then describe in language their feelings about dying, as does Lerner. He considers the thoughts of philosophers and poets about death, muses about his own death and his wish to see the dramas of his family members' lives and his world play out. But when a person is actually in the throes of death, when his or her body is wracked by pain, language ceases to be a possibility. People who are dying may utter random words or sounds devoid of meaning—a cry, a moan, or a shriek—or reach the point of silence. For this reason we have no description from a person who is dying of what this experience is actually like. At best we can observe the dying body.

Nonetheless, descriptions of the dying or dead body can be powerfully evocative. Such descriptions depend on the images created by words and not the words themselves to convey a feeling about death. For example, Anatole Broyard offers this poignant description of his father dying of prostate cancer: "his hands in the air that day, immobile as death, and excruciatingly cramped in the act of sculpting a likeness of his pain."[103] Yet, his father's dying, in all its heartbreak, is barely noticed by those around him: no one in the ward paid the slightest attention to "those hands, which ought to have conducted the orchestrated empathy of every living soul in sight."[104] Robert Lipsyte offers a similarly powerful description of his adult son at the bed of his mother who has just died, his arms wrapped around her legs as he sobs. Not the words, but the image the words create, suggests emotions that lie beyond words. As with the pietà, the representation of the body in the posture of sorrow evokes the wrenching sense of loss at the death of a loved one.[105]

Ultimately, in the face of death, all language gives way to silence. Lerner comments about his own writing and immortality, suggesting that his writing might provide a "wisp of mortality" in the guise of a student here or there who might pick up one of his books.[106] But he knows that his voice will become faint and eventually disappear. Harold Brodkey continues to write close to his death but acknowledges that what he is recording, while he still can, is his own disappearance. "And I am still writing, as you see. I am practicing making entries in my journal, recording my passage into nonexistence. This identity, this mind, this particular cast of speech, is nearly over."[107]

As these writers struggle to find language for their pain and suffering we learn a great deal not only about their difficulty in communicating but also about the nature of illness. As Scarry makes so clear, the pain of one person is not readily accessible to another. Words fail in the face of suffering. Language intrudes itself between the sufferer and the listener, creating a distance from the felt experience. Frustrated in their attempts to find language, writers resort to quoting biblical and literary passages to express their feelings. Or they speak of illness in metaphorical terms. Sometimes they simply give up. Yet in the very act of struggling with language they do something important—they bring us into experience of frustration, loneliness, and futility that the ill and injured feel when they cannot communicate. They acquaint us with the limitations that are part of the human condition. And, at moments, they soar beyond those limits by the very act of putting into words this very experience of limitation.

— CHAPTER V —

Narrative Form

*But as we examine definitions and redefinitions of self emerging
from victim narratives, we must keep in mind that each one of them
represents a combat, more often than not unconscious, between fragment
and form, disaster and intactness, birdsong and pandemonium.*
—Lawrence Langer, *Holocaust Testimonies.*

Why do I think of things falling apart? Were they ever whole?
—Arthur Miller, *After the Fall.*

Just as writers struggle to find language to describe the experience of
illness or injury, they search for ways to tell their story that capture
the temporary or permanent disruption or break that illness or accident causes in their lives. Some resist telling a linear story and instead
write essays or a narrative that is itself more circular or multilayered.
Most, however, end up employing the straightforward linear narrative in which we generally tell stories. They recount the series of
events that followed one upon the other—the accident or diagnosis,
the meetings with doctors, the treatments, and finally the restoration
to health or the acceptance of death.

Yet in the end even those who write a linear narrative often end
up joining with those who reject it in pointing out the limits of a linear story for representing illness and disability. They argue that the
linear narrative, structured around a beginning, middle, and end,
inevitably carries the plot along from crisis to resolution. Serious illness or disability, on the other hand, because it has an indeterminate
beginning and an unknown ending, is not adequately served by a linear narrative. While the story can and often is told chronologically,
the real focus of an illness story is on the ill person's internal experience as it unfolds outside time. What the author of an illness story

attempts to explain, alongside the unfolding of events in chronological time, is that a more fractured internal experience is occurring.

The frustration writers of illness narratives feel with this form, or sometimes with any form, leads many to diverge from their story to actually discuss the question of narrative form. While these discussions might seem esoteric in the middle of these stories, they are significant in that they reflect the writers' continued struggle to find a way to adequately describe their experience.

Within their narratives these writers consider the overall shape of their narrative in relationship to the condition of their ill or disabled body; they question the very act of writing a coherent story about life coming apart; they wonder how to represent the parts of their experience during which they were unconscious, medicated, or simply disconnected from life. Their concern is with how best to represent what is chaotic, broken or multilayered in their experience. Essentially they grapple with the fundamental question at the heart of an illness narrative: how to represent the experience of serious damage to the body and self and of major disruption in a life. What they discern in the process is that their wish to represent the truth of how shattering illness is conflicts with their desire to bestow coherence on that experience.

These discussions of form, therefore, while literary, are essentially attempts to come to terms with the chaotic, fractured, nonlinear nature of the illness experience. Writers confront the same problem with form they encountered with language: the available forms seem inadequate for representing the experience. And yet their search for an appropriate form, much like their search for descriptive language, opens the way to a greater understanding of the nature of serious illness and its tendency to defy expression. By inviting us to reflect on the disruptive nature of illness and how difficult it is to shape that experience into a story without betraying its reality, these writers move us toward a new story of illness whose message will be of value in our larger culture: illness confounds us, is bigger than we are, and often refuses to be managed.

The desire to tell an illness story can arise from different motivations. Most people wish to impose on their experience both order and meaning. As Arthur Kleinman says, "The illness narrative is a story the patient tells . . . to give coherence to the distinctive events and long-term course of suffering. The plot lines, core metaphors, and rhetorical devices that structure the illness narrative are drawn from cultural and personal models for arranging experiences in meaningful ways and for effectively communicating those meanings."[1] But some wonder if this imposition of coherence negates or downplays how devastating the lived experience is and how severe the damage done to the self and body can be. They wish to describe the disruption of illness as much as impose order on it. I would suggest that the best storytellers are successfully able to hold in tension these two different and seemingly contradictory purposes at the heart of illness narration—to represent the devastation of the experience and to transform the raw and shattered experience into a story with shape and coherence.

The wish to represent the lived experience gives rise to some recurrent and perplexing questions about narrative. Should the body of the narrative mirror the lived experience of illness and itself be shattered or broken? If that is possible within a linear narrative, what would it look like? If not, what would be an alternative form in which to capture the circularity and disrupted nature of a life with illness? Finally, does the very act of writing itself, apart from the choice of form, bestow a continuity, coherence, and directionality not present in the lived experience? These questions lead writers to confront a general, philosophical problem—that in many ways the nature of illness and the nature of narrative are diametrically opposed: to be ill is to be disrupted; to write is to bestow order.

Chaos versus Coherence

Both Charles Mee and Leonard Kriegel come to reflect on these questions of form. Each is aware that polio damaged his body and disrupted his life in ways that one never completely recovers from. Yet at the same time each embraces the idea that narrative can help to lend coherence to that experience.

Because polio damaged his body and threw his life into chaos, Mee considers the possibility that a more fractured narrative might be appropriate. The form of *Woyzeck*, a play by Georg Buchner, captures for Mee something of what it is like to live in a crippled body: "a play whose scenes break off suddenly in midsentence, where bits of scenes occur out of place, inexplicable things happen; a play composed of chunks and shards, broken pieces, raw, awkward, clumsy, with events crashing into one another without reason or cause; a shattered world, fucked up and roughhewn."[2] Mee notices that what he admires—that the playwright resists the logical sequence and causality that characterize linear narrative—is rejected by many directors who impose on these fragments a logical order. "They remove the chunks of broken, pointless scenes; they make a more logical order of what remains, they put in transitions from one moment to the next, they smooth it out, they make it 'work.' In short, they kill it."[3] And in the process they deprive the audience of the feeling of randomness and brokenness.

As a playwright, Mee wants to write such disrupted plays: "I really don't want to write well-made sentences and paragraphs, narratives that flow, structures that have a sense of wholeness and balance, books that feel intact. Intact people should write intact books with sound narratives built of sound paragraphs that unfold with a sense of dependable cause and effect, solid structures you can rely on."[4] He argues for a narrative form that represents life as out of control and a plot that moves in all directions, since he himself cannot walk in a straight line; a play full of violent action, like a car crashing out of control, that would better embody the experience of having one's life shattered in a flash. "To me, sentences should veer and smash up, career out of control; get under way and find themselves unable to stop, switch directions suddenly and irrevocably, break off, come to a sighing inconclusiveness."[5]

As Mee puts it elsewhere, "If a writer's writings constitute a 'body of work,' then my body of work, to feel true to me, must feel fragmented."[6] Nonetheless, it is equally important to Mee to impose some kind of coherence on that experience. Mee admires the ability of the Greeks to represent the truth and even the chaos and brutality of life while also making something beautiful and whole of it. This is what he tries to do in his plays. He will take the text of a classic Greek play, "smash it to ruins, and then, atop of its ruined structure of plot and character, write a new play, with all-new language, characters of today speaking like people of today."[7]

Interestingly, Mee writes the story of his own life in the form of a conventional linear narrative. Within that form he movingly describes the disruption by polio in his life. But he also partakes of the benefits of chronology and a consistent voice and point of view to bestow order on the events of his childhood. It is within this coherent, organized, and aesthetically pleasing whole that he talks about, rather than enacts, the fragmentation of his experience. Mee recognizes that his desire for coherence is as strong as his wish to represent chaos. He paraphrases the physician Eric Cassell: "Every life . . . has a sense of wholeness or correctness, of fitness and cogency, that is made up of the remembered common past of the family, of the web of friendships and relationships, of expectations and hopes for the future that inform the present, of the unconscious dreams and fears, of the continuously rewritten autobiography we all carry with us in our minds; and all of these are subject to damage."[8] He goes on: "The aesthetic whole of a life must be reconstructed if a person is to regain a sense of coherence."[9]

There remains the question of whether or how well one can ever represent a shattering experience. Perhaps Mee could have chosen a different form that would have better reflected or embodied the damage he experienced. Would it have been accessible or of interest to the reader? Or would the reader have felt deprived of the coherence he or she somehow desired? I would argue that with regard to the story of illness and injury, a representation of the catastrophic nature of these experiences, while it may reflect the fact that illness by its very nature is disruptive, leaves us without the resolution we desire. If, however, the writer offers a coherent narrative, there remains the equally unsatisfying reality that something of the rawness of the experience is lost.

In his essay "Falling into Life" Leonard Kriegel suggests that narrative offers him genuine possibilities for lending coherence, particularly symmetry, to his life experience. As a crippled man whose gait is awkward and body assymetrical, he longs for symmetry and sees writing as a way for him to symbolically reconstitute himself: "I am possessed by a peculiar passion: I want to believe that my life has been balanced out."[10] Kriegel chooses the less structured form of an essay because it allows him to digress from a chronological telling of his story to structure his experience differently. Within his essays he counterposes parallel experiences as a way to achieve symmetry. As I noted earlier, he describes three instances of falling that represent critical moments in his life: as a crippled boy he had to learn to fall to avoid hurting himself; as a middle-aged man to accept help when he fell and depend on friends; and as an older man to accept that he will fall into death.

Elsewhere Kriegel counterposes the devastation of polio with the fulfillment he has achieved in his life. He recalls sitting in a café in Paris in 1965, separated from his wife and two-year-old son with whom he'd been living in Holland where he was a Fulbright lecturer. He was overwhelmed by a feeling of loneliness and a sense of loss: "I suddenly gasped, stifling a sob as if I had been hit in the solar plexus and could feel myself doubling over. The reality I had lived with for twenty-one years had once again overwhelmed me. *I was a cripple.* And I missed the legs I had lost to a polio virus. . . . The loss of my legs enraged me: It would always enrage me. And I would never get used to it. Its arbitrariness, its naked proclamation of what I could and could not do, of what I could never again do."[11] Yet, he explains, his rage is always counterpoised with a pride in his accomplishments. He recalls walking in the Tuileries with his wife and son three weeks earlier; his son, grasping a finger of the hand with which Kriegel holds his crutch, "walked as proudly as any other two-year-old moving along with his father."[12]

In their narratives Mee and Kriegel describe their shattered experience but ultimately do not embody it, perhaps for good reason. A more direct representation of chaos, unmediated by an author who reflects on and organizes experience, is not often successful. Arthur Frank makes this point when he identifies a group of illness stories he calls chaos stories: they are written during a crisis or as if during a crisis when the experience is raw; they are without logical sequence and associative or causal links. The "plot imagines life never getting better. Stories are chaotic in their absence of narrative order. Events are told as the storyteller experiences life: without sequence or discernible causality."[13] Frank argues that it is actually impossible to write a chaos story, that such chaos is the opposite of story. At best, he suggests, we can record the voice of someone speaking while in a chaotic situation. He offers the example of a woman with a chronic illness trying to describe her mother, who has Alzheimer's disease. She says, "And if I'm trying to get dinner ready and I'm already feeling bad, she's in front of the refrigerator. Then she goes to put her hand on the stove and I got the fire on. And then she's in front of the microwave and then she's in front of the silverware drawer. And— and if I send her out she gets mad at me. And then it's awful. That's when I have a really, a really bad time."[14] Paradoxically, this passage, although a record of this woman's exact speech, actually fails to capture the feeling of chaos. And it leaves us feeling irritated. Even what Frank calls "the incessant present" that characterizes the speaker's report fails to create immediacy.[15] Without a speaker or writer to transform the experience into something coherent enough to be communicated, we are left, ironically, with a verbal chaos that fails to communicate the feel of chaos.

A successful representation of chaos requires not only a skilled and disciplined writer but also, paradoxically, some distance from the chaotic experience. Only then does the writer have enough control of language and form to communicate what is devastating about an experience. This issue is addressed in a review of an exhibit on Anne Frank's writing. Elizabeth Becker, reporting on the exhibit, suggests that Anne Frank's diary has lived on in the public's imagination while hundreds of other diaries have not precisely because she, even while living in hiding, achieves enough distance from the experience to concentrate on crafting her writing.[16] As Klaus Muller, the co-curator of the exhibit points out, Anne wrote in detail about her daily life and her hopes for the future and then rewrote pages of her diary everyday, while also reading and collecting quotes from the great writers she was reading. Those who are successful in writing a story of illness that captures the chaotic aspect of the experience are not simply pouring their raw thoughts onto the page; they are struggling with language and form to communicate what often feels formless and overwhelming. It is the writer's discipline that provides access to what is chaotic.

Linear Narrative

Those writers who struggle specifically with the question of linear narrative recognize that the form itself provides a kind of comfort that perhaps works against a true representation of a shattering experience. They sense what Lawrence Langer so beautifully explored in his book: "Written memoirs, by the very strategies available to their authors—style, chronology, analogy, imagery, dialogue, a sense of character, a coherent moral vision—strive to narrow this space, easing us into their unfamiliar world through familiar (and hence comforting?) literary devices."[17] Elsewhere Langer points out that "a written narrative is finished when we begin to read it, its opening, middle and end are already established between the covers of the book. This *appearance* of form is re-assuring."[18] Ultimately, the author who wishes to communicate what is unsettling about an experience must face this fact that the use of literary devices in itself is comforting.

A writer can hardly refrain from using literary devices, however. Nor can the writer really escape linearity. In his essay "Tales Told by a Computer," Tim Parks suggests that even when a novelist deviates from linearity by starting in the middle or at the end, "over the trajectory of the work as a whole, the reader expects a chronology of a kind to be reconstructed."[19] Even writers like Joyce or Borges who choose a nonchronological ordering of events cannot ultimately escape linearity. The fact "that one reads a book from front to back accepting whatever ordering of events the author chooses" is a submission to chronology. As Parks succinctly puts it, "A desire to be outside time, free from linearity, can only be expressed within time." Besides, Parks suggests, "much of the pathos of our lives has to do with the stark simplicity of chronology: birth, youth, maturity, death."[20]

Sometimes a writer's discussion of form rather that actual choice of a form focuses the reader on the multilayered and complex nature of experience. Floyd Skloot explains that he has come to prefer long poems because they can hold a certain tension and embody an internal looseness that better reflects the nature of lived experience, in his case, chronic fatigue syndrome. He discusses two musical pieces by Franz Schubert that, like the short and long poem, represent different possibilities for depicting life experience. The first, "Die Fore-leg," is a song based on a short poem about the catching of trout. Skloot describes it as characterized by "charm and whimsy, not moral lessons."[21] It holds the possibility of depicting life in an uncompli-cated way. The longer *Trout* Quintet that Schubert wrote two years later includes an extended set of variations on the original tune. Skloot finds this longer form allows for different moods, pacing, har-monies, and, significantly, discordant notes, and can therefore better express the complexity of a life with serious illness. "In the amplitude of a longer work, there is sweetness, to be sure, loving duets in the strings, gently flowing passages for the piano, frolicsome melodies. But there is also moroseness, hectic interludes, sudden shifts in char-acter that shatter the calm."[22]

Skloot later explains that the complexity of music provided him with a way to understand that his "body's symphony now included a long movement of pure chaos, somber and discordant, but one that would lead somewhere worth going if I learned to listen."[23] In the introduction to her memoir *Zeno's Paradox*, Victoria Bell similarly considers the fugue a form preferable to the linear narrative to describe her experience with lymphoma.[24] "Recently I have realized that what I previously regarded as a linear progression toward 'truth' resembles a spiral rather than a straight line. Might it not be better if I could convert the story into a massive fugue where layers inter-weave and the sum is never reducible to its parts?"[25]

Linear versus Circular Narrative

Georgina Kleege chooses a nonlinear form to discuss the experience of blindness. She believes that linear narratives, "structured around conflict, epiphany, and resolution . . . promote the notion that blind-ness is something one either triumphs over or is defeated by."[26] She therefore forgoes a chronological narrative and instead writes about blindness itself. She discusses the cultural aspects of blindness, the visual experience of someone with severely impaired sight, and the experience of reading. As she puts it, "Although the sequence of these chapters is not chronological, the arrangement of material maps a thought process. This process is cyclical rather than linear. It spirals around its subject in ever-smaller circles."[27] Her personal experience serves primarily to illustrate a point about blindness. For example, she describes a conversation she had with her father while standing very close to a painting in the Museum of Modern Art in New York City not so much to tell her story as to share her thoughts about eye contact, to describe the pain around her eyes, and finally to explain her decision to use Braille as an aid.

John Hull also argues that the linear narrative forces the writer to present blindness as a problem to be resolved. Like Kleege he experiences his blindness as an ongoing part of his life. Yet his experience is different from Kleege's. Whereas Kleege lived most of her life as blind, Hull became blind in his forties. For him, consequently, blindness was a devastating experience that radically changed his life and entailed an enormous sense of loss. Hull finds that those autobiographies that depict blind people as stoic and resigned gloss over the damage done by the experience. Like Kleege, he also finds that what he calls "literary accounts" demand a particular structure that fails to represent the disrupted and continuing difficulty of his experience. As he noted, "They had a beginning, a middle and an end. They were like novels, with an interesting style, a climax or a resolution."[28]

Hull writes a different kind of book. Although in his introduction he provides a chronological summary of his life—the situation of his parents, his birth, his gradual and then total loss of eyesight—most of the book consists of dated entries, much like a diary. The book grows out of recordings he made over a three-year period of his thoughts, feelings, opinions, and struggles related to his blindness. He talks about his children, work, relationships, and dreams in a way that, he argues, would not be possible in a strictly linear narrative: he works from inside the experience in an attempt to remain true to how it felt rather than imposing a linear structure on it. He explains that for this reason his "book is not tightly organized. There are bits and pieces all over the place. There are times when solutions seem to be in sight, so to speak, but there are continual relapses, when nothing seems to have been gained or learned." Of course in the hands of a less skilled writer the work might simply seemed disorganized or incoherent. Hull goes on, "If there is repetition, it is because the same problems and the same experiences went round and round, interpreted from many aspects."[29] In place of narrative progression there is circularity; in place of continuity there are breaks and diversions; in place of resolution there is an open-ended conclusion. The form he chooses allows him to describe in considerable depth the difficulties the loss of his eyesight caused in his life.

Hull, however, does not do himself justice when he describes his book as "all over the place." The book traces an associative rather than a chronological journey and ultimately records the process through which he attempts to find a sense of coherence in his life. Believing that "a unified life is superior to a fragmented life," he understands that it must be a unity that includes losses.[30] "I will be all the more sane if I have been able to accept, to include, to harmonize more and more of my experience."[31] But he believes, in fact, that even his blindness must take its rightful place among other parts of his life. "My overriding attempt must be to have the courage to be faithful as a whole, that is, as a person in whose life this is one aspect amongst many others."[32] As a religious person he goes on to say that his own life must be seen as part of a larger whole.

The circular rather than linear nature of illness and disability is equally characteristic of grief. In his book *A Grief Observed* C. S. Lewis captures the circular nature of the grief he felt at the death of his wife, Helen Joy Gresham.[33] Lewis had married Gresham, a woman with whom he shared a rich intellectual life, knowing that she was dying of cancer. After her death Lewis finds himself returning again and again to the raw and inconsolable feeling of grief. He describes a night sometime after his wife's death when "all the hells of young grief have opened again; the mad words, the bitter resentment, the fluttering in the stomach, the nightmare unreality, the wallowed-in tears."[34] He is struck by the fact that he never seems to move past these feelings. "One keeps on emerging from a phase, but it always recurs. Round and round. Everything repeats. Am I going in circles, or dare I hope I am on a spiral? But if a spiral, am I going up or down it?"[35] He captures this even more poignantly by comparing it to physical pain. "The same leg is cut off time after time. The first plunge of the knife into the flesh is felt again and again."[36]

Gaps in Experience

How does a person describe the gaps in experience caused by illness or accident? Writers employ various devices to represent the gaps and interruptions caused by unconsciousness from disease, medication, or coma. And, as we saw in chapter 3, a number of writers describe the efforts they made in their lives to establish continuity where there had been or would be a break. Middlebrook gathers the recollections of others to reconstruct her experience during her bone marrow transplant; after his stroke Robert McCrum resumes the ordinary activities of life to connect his new life with his old; Gilda Radner runs a videotape of herself playing tennis so others can hold a sense of her life as continuous.

Some writers use narrative itself not just to represent the gap but to bridge it. Richard Seltzer writes *Raising the Dead*, the story of his recovery from Legionnaires' disease, for example, in the main as an attempt to fill in the gap in his experience caused by coma. He actually tries to narrate his experience during the twenty-three days he was in a coma and the time after he emerged when he was in a psychotic state as the result of his withdrawal from medication. To do so, he invents a shadow narrator who is also himself, but who speaks in the third person about what is going on in the unconscious Seltzer. This shadow narrator is beside the bed of the patient, Seltzer, and comments, "I, the author, am also there standing, or rather, hovering bodiless above and to the side, out of the way yet able to see, to hear, now and then able to reach down if I wish and touch him."37 As this narrator he will continue to speak in the third person about himself, the patient in the coma, until he emerges from the coma and can speak for himself. From this imagined position, as himself outside himself, he describes himself in the bed as "little more than a skeleton."

The shadow narrator device works well enough when he describes what he observes about the patient in the bed—how he looks, moves, and sounds, but it feels contrived when this shadow narrator begins to describe the patient's internal experience, particularly his hallucinations. Using the records of his hallucinations that Seltzer's nurses and family kept, Seltzer has this shadow narrator tell the reader where the patient's imagination roams during the night: "In the course of a single night he travels to a medieval monastery in 13th-century Ireland, where he undergoes a harsh novitiate. . . . Minutes later he is in the delta of the river Nile, wading among the fat, yellowish serpents that are native to the region. From there, it is on to Molokai on a tall sailing ship. Father Damien himself comes out to greet him."[38] While the narration accurately represents the content of the hallucinations, it fails to communicate the feel of them. It is, in fact, impossible to know what Seltzer experienced while he was hallucinating. Whether Seltzer's intention is to shed light on the experience of coma or demonstrate literary innovation, he leaves the reader too busy trying to figure out what is going on. And he fails, understandably, to inform us of what the experience of unconsciousness is like.

Serious illness creates other kinds of gaps in a life that writers struggle to represent. Pain, for example, can be so intense that it removes a person from active participation in life. Is there a way to represent this withdrawal from life? Few writers have been very successful. The present-day enthusiasm for Alphonse Daudet's notes results in part from the fact that as a form the notes do successfully suggest the gaps in his life caused by suffering. Ironically, Daudet had no interest in his notes as a form for representing the gaps in his experience; it is contemporary readers who have come to admire the way the breaks suggest absence due to suffering. As Julian Barnes suggests, the notes "seem an appropriate form in which to deal with one's dying."[39] He points out that the set, "though organized, and with a certain inevitable plot-progression, remains a collection of notes; but this isn't necessarily a disadvantage."[40] As Barnes suggests, "They imply the time, and suffering, which elapses between each being made: here is a decade or so of torment reduced to fifty pages."[41] The sentences that break off, the lapses between entries, and the sparseness of the notes all suggest to the reader something of the disrupted nature of Daudet's life.

In reading Daudet's notes we actually experience interruption. We cannot help but be aware that Daudet, the narrator, is struggling with his disease even as he writes. There are breaks that imply Daudet is too sick to write. Time stops, and Daudet is so absorbed in his body that there is no world outside. As we read along, perhaps expecting the kind of continuity that characterizes most stories, we feel the continuity being repeatedly broken. The thoughts are short, succinct, and undeveloped. Although at times Daudet describes his suffering, we have the feeling that the real pain exists outside the text; its best expression is absence and silence. The notes are a remarkable and rare example of a form that manages to communicate this silence.

Interestingly, Daudet, somewhat like Seltzer, struggles with what kind of narrator can represent the internal experience of suffering. He also struggles with his own internal conflict about whether to reveal his suffering to his family. He is caught between his felt need to express the truth about his suffering and his wish to do so in an artistic form that would protect his family from a full knowledge of his suffering. On the one hand Daudet declines to write a novel because it would not be a truthful rendition of his experience. On the other hand, he rejects the possibility of autobiography, even if published posthumously, because he was not interested in writing what he called a "testament of complaint against my family."[42] In addition, in nineteenth-century France such personal and revealing writing was generally confined to diaries or private correspondence.

As Barnes relates, Daudet was very excited when he worked out a solution to his dilemma. Daudet imagines writing a dialogue between two men who are ill and in pain, each of whom represents a side of Daudet's internal conflict. One who is single can express all his feelings without fear of hurting his family. This was important to Daudet. As he touchingly puts it, "If you've got small children, you don't want to spoil the few happy, innocent hours of their lives, leaving them with the memory of an old dad who was always moaning and complaining."[43] The other man who is married cannot complain but can receive the comfort from family that he would lack were he single.

Would Daudet's dialogue actually have worked? It is doubtful that these characters would have communicated the emotional immediacy of his notes. More likely these characters, envisioned in the notes not as living people but as embodiments of two sides of an intellectual conflict, would seem wooden and their discussion too intellectual, although in Daudet's hands they might have come to life. At the very least this imagined dialogue would have explained his dilemma about how to express his pain while sparing his family.

Nancy Mairs, in an essay entitled "On Living Behind Bars," simply explains that there will be gaps in the story of her experience. She explains that the narrative she is writing of the six months she spent at Metropolitan State Hospital in Waltham, Massachusetts, in treatment for depression and anxiety "will be full of such gaps and lapses, because during the latter part of my story my brain was zapped twenty-one times."[44] "Electroshock treatments left her with little memory of that time, mostly random images, some in remarkable detail and clarity, but few embedded in any logically continuous context."[45] She uses the analogy of a person restringing a broken necklace to describe how one deals with gaps in conscious experience and to represent how a life can be reconstructed as a whole even when parts of that life experience have been lost. "I had once, many years later, a string of black, clay Mexican beads on a nylon thread that snapped suddenly, in the middle of a class I was teaching, scattering little fish and birds and balls every which way." Her students gathered up what pieces they could, and her "foster son restrung them, in a new pattern necessitated by the missing pieces, into a shorter necklace. One can, to some extent, recover one's losses, but the bits that roll under the shelves, into the corners, out the door are gone for good."[46]

Interruption

In a linear narrative transitions keep the story moving but thereby eliminate the interruptions characteristic of a life with illness.[47] Virginia Woolf pursues the theme of illness as interruption in her essay "On Being Ill." In the oft-quoted opening passage Woolf wonders why illness has not become one of the great subjects of literature, given all it reveals about life and experience and given that even the most mundane experience of bodily affliction throws us "into the pit of death."[48] She ends her list of the kinds of intense experiences illness entails by referring to what it's like to be at the dentist and wake up and hear him say, "Rinse the mouth—rinse the mouth."[49] By interrupting her own eloquent litany with a reminder to the reader of the banal and ignoble nature of the body's afflictions, here dental afflictions, Woolf actually captures the way in which the demands of the body are insistent. This first paragraph of Woolf's essay, then, with its description of interruption, foreshadows the final story in her essay.

That story, retold by Woolf, is taken from popular literature and used to demonstrate how death can brutally interrupt even the most carefree life. Woolf purports to entertain the reader with a discussion of how illness gives people permission to read literature generally considered frivolous, like Augustus Hare's *The Story of Two Noble Lives*, a story of two nineteenth-century aristocratic ladies.[50] But in no way is Woolf's intention to consider the possibilities of frivolous literature; rather, she turns this notion on its head to reveal this is a story of death and grief. Woolf pulls the reader in by describing in detail the plot in a way that suggests it is a predictable story that will end happily ever after. It is a story of English aristocrats, parties, marriages, castles, trips abroad, lovely daughters dancing and sketching. At the center of it is Lady Waterford, who busies herself with entertaining and charity and bids her husband good-bye when he goes off hunting. But then Woolf shocks the reader. Lady Waterford "would wave to him and think each time, what if this should be the last? And so it was, that winter's morning."[51] Into this lively, everyday scene in a frivolous story Woolf introduces death. She ends the essay with two striking images noted by Sir John Leslie, a character in the story: one of Lady Waterford standing at the window as the hearse pulled away and the other, after the funeral: "The curtain, heavy, mid-Victorian, plush perhaps . . . was all crushed together where she had grasped it in her agony."[52] This final image of Lady Waterford grasping the curtain suggests that any moment death can interrupt life.

Donald Hall intends his book *Life Work* to be about his life as a writer, but it also becomes a book about the way illness interrupts a writer's life.[53] The first half is about Hall's intended subject—the nature of a writer's work life, his own and others. He roams freely from descriptions of his ancestors' work to his own teaching and writing, from a discussion of attitudes toward work to dictionary definitions of work. He discusses Henry Moore's work, ballplayers' work, his everyday work, and what constitutes a good workday or a bad one.

The second half is a description of how his work life is interrupted by illness and the prospect of death. Hall begins with the moment of interruption in his own life. Celebrating with his wife, Jane Kenyon, who has just been awarded a Guggenheim fellowship for her poetry, he is interrupted by a call from his internist with news that his CEA (a blood protein that marks carcinoma) count is very high. A scan indicates that the colon cancer for which he had been treated earlier had metastasized to his liver. The best outcome of surgery would be a return to an ordinary life interrupted regularly by three month checkups; the worst that he would die.

In this second half of the book Hall's focus changes. He now writes as someone aware that he is living an interrupted life and writing an interrupted book. He explains the way appointments, tests, and surgery interrupt his routine. He longs to return to his writing projects, but work is interrupted by tasks such as writing "letters canceling dates and postponing interviews" because of his upcoming surgery.[54] Although his style is casual and talky, his writing is interrupted at points and often abruptly by thoughts of death. Sometimes Hall narrates these interruptions in his thought. For example, while he is describing a particular work project the thought of cancer intrudes. "I've proofread *Their Ancient Glittering Eyes* again, and it looks clean. Like the left lobe of a liver?"[55]

Many more times Hall tells us of returning to his work, making plans, only to have them interrupted by illness or thoughts of illness. Before his operation, he writes, "I have a list of topics to keep me busy. The alternative is tears, appropriate enough but miserable."[56] His planning of topics is interrupted by his thoughts about death. "I keep thinking of Jane, of my mother, of my children and grandchildren. I'm not exactly afraid but I am surely *sad*."[57] Sometimes these intrusive thoughts about illness are not momentary but persistent, comprising a kind of shadow experience. Letters from friends about his manuscripts take him "back inside my poems and away from my damned liver—but memory of that dark hourglass barbell shape reruns itself on the witless screen. I try to snow it over: *Go away, go away, go away*."[58]

Hall is intrigued by artists who refuse to have their work interrupted even by the persistent demands of illness. He describes how Henry James continued to write despite age, illness, physical and mental breakdowns. After his second stroke, his thoughts confused, James continued to dictate to his helper, "riding on grooves established by sixty years of sentences in the morning . . . making the clauses of his adult style."[59] But, as Hall points out, although the form survives, his clauses are devoid of reason. He quotes a passage from James: "We simply shift nursling of genius from one maternal breast to the other and the trick is played, the false not averted. . . . Astounding little stepchild of God's astounding young stepmother! . . . five miles off at the renewed affronts that we see coming from the great, and that we know they will accept. The fault is that they had found themselves too easily great, and the effect of that, definitely, had been, within them, the want of long provision for it."[60] Hall comments that "the work survives the worker: Henry Moore without memory sketching in a wheelchair, Henry James on the bed of paralysis speaking a senseless syntax."[61] But he leaves us to wonder what it means that the work survives. After all, James's sentences no longer make sense.

In a sense Hall manages to write a book that holds the tension between his knowing he may die sooner than expected and his desire to go on living and working. He finds a form that embodies his living and his dying—a memoir of work in which he describes and enacts both the way illness interrupts his life as well as the way he goes on with his life and work. He writes a narrative that contains the breaks, diversions, and interruptions in his life. He gives the reader the feeling of how life is interrupted and how the possibility of death intrudes and is interwoven into a life. His narrative is the coherent whole that contains within it the holes, breaks, and diversions that illness causes in a life.

These writers, then, are grappling with the limits and possibilities of narrative form for representing the experience of illness. Some writers, finding that certain forms, particularly the linear narrative, fail to represent the disrupted, chaotic nature of the illness experience, search for other ways to represent how illness and injury interrupt the continuity of life or leave gaps in a person's consciousness or memory. Although a few experiment with different forms in an attempt to actually represent the experience of interruption, their attempts are often not successful. Others focus on how, whatever the limits of a particular form, the creation of a narrative can lend coherence to a chaotic experience; telling a story even becomes a way of symbolically reconstituting a sense of self. By filling in the gaps, making transitions between events, imposing a logical sequence and arranging incidents in a particular way, the storyteller reestablishes continuity with a former life or creates a new kind of continuity.

What becomes clear in reading these narratives is that the capacity of narrative to bestow order and meaning on experience is both its limitation and its possibility. A narrative structure that irons out the disorder fails to represent the rawness of experience and, with regard to illness, the extent of the damage caused to the self and to a life. Yet even those writers intent on representing this damage still value the capacity of narrative to lend coherence to their chaotic experience. The best writers, I would suggest, manage to acknowledge the limits of narrative while partaking of its benefits.

— CHAPTER VI —

Endings

If you want a happy ending, that depends, of course,
on where you stop the story.

—Orson Welles

When Primo Levi threw himself down a stairwell in 1987, people refused to believe he had committed suicide. Although his books on the Holocaust were deeply disturbing in their depiction of the unimaginable horror played out daily in the concentration camp at Auschwitz, his story was generally read as a triumph narrative, that is, as a testament to Levi's ability to survive even the most devastating and unspeakable treatment. Perhaps because people needed Levi to be a symbol of hope, they could not accept the possibility that he committed suicide.

Reading in the *New York Times* an account of a symposium of writers and scholars discussing Levi and his work, William Styron was "fascinated but, finally, appalled" at the participants' refusal to accept Levi's suicide. "It was as if this man whom they had all so greatly admired, and who had endured so much at the hands of the Nazis—a man of exemplary resilience and courage—had by his suicide demonstrated a frailty, a crumbling of character."[1] It was in response to this article and to what he considered widespread public denial of the seriousness of Levi's despair that Styron was uncharacteristically moved to write personally about his own depression in a *New York Times* op-ed piece and then his book *Darkness Visible.* Given that, in his opinion, "the pain of severe depression is quite unimaginable to those who have not suffered it, and it kills in many instances because its anguish can no longer be borne,"[2] he took it upon himself to inform people of the seriousness and life-threatening

/ *119* /

nature of depression. He saw the public's insistence on a happy ending as arising from a lack of knowledge of depression's reality.

We all find particularly disturbing the notion that a person might not recover from physical or emotional illness. If recovery is not possible, we at least desire that a person make peace with his or her situation. And yet this is not always what happens. As many narrators of serious illness acknowledge, they cannot assure the reader they are recovered and, as some admit, they still find it difficult to accept what has happened to them. Even if their future health looks promising, a happy ending that does not acknowledge the difficulty of accepting one's mortality seems inappropriate for an illness story.

Of course the range of endings is as broad as the range of illnesses and injuries. In cases of acute illness where health is restored the author can write a happy ending without betraying the truth of his or her experience. Even when cure is likely though uncertain, the writer can end with some resolution, perhaps acknowledging that the ending is unknown, as Musa Mayer does in her memoir about her breast cancer, *Examining Myself*: "This book is difficult for me to end, for the ending is still open, the future unknown. But that's a fact of life with which we all contend. . . . Although I have not recaptured my former self, physically or emotionally, I do feel recovered."[3] But with illnesses that recur, injuries that cause permanent damage, chronic illness, or even with acute illness where anxiety and fear remain, the narrator often wants to communicate that the end does not mean resolution. Aware of their mortality, perhaps still suffering from their malady or facing death, many writers struggle to find an ending that remains true to the unpredictable or sorrowful reality of their situation.

In reading illness stories I discovered that a number of writers end their stories in a way that is confused but fascinating: they offer one ending and then critique it, rewrite it, and even rewrite it again. I also realized that the ending of my own memoir exhibits exactly this kind of complication if not confusion, as I will explain later. Whether intentionally or not, many of us embody in our endings our difficulty dealing with the unknown future or complex nature of our situation. These renegotiated endings deserve attention because they are critical to understanding the intractability of the illness story. In terms of content they underscore the fact that no one who is ill simply assumes a happy ending. In terms of form, these confused endings reflect the inadequacy of the triumph narrative as a form for representing illness. With serious illness the fact that the author does not have control of the ending clashes with his or her need to put closure on the story. Here the writer faces most starkly the fact that writing does not bestow immortality.

In the preceding chapter I considered the story Virginia Woolf tells at the end of her essay "On Being Ill" to demonstrate how she suggests the feeling of interruption that illness or death causes. That story is also interesting for its ending. The way Woolf recounts this story of two aristocratic Victorian women leads us to expect the happy ending of a Victorian romance, but she resists a romantic ending and, in fact, shocks us by ending with a death. Similarly, Jill Ker Conway recounts her conscious choice to resist the pressure to offer a happy or romantic ending to her book *The Road to Coorain*.[4] Written explicitly as an alternative to stories about the Australian outback that are centered on the myth of the heroic natural man, Conway ends the story of her life in the outback—a woman's story in a woman's voice—at the point when she leaves Australia, not two years later, when she gets married. She explains her non-Shakespearean choice to resist ending with a wedding as her attempt to prevent her readers from resting with an easy, stereotypical sense that she simply settled into family life.[5] This is what Woolf is doing when she ends the romance of aristocratic ladies with a death. And it is also what Donald Hall does when he ends his book *Life Work* before he receives the test results that will give him a sense of whether he will die sooner or later.

This kind of conscious attempt to resist the happy ending characterizes the conclusion of many books about illness aside from those of the triumphal school. But it is often not a smooth attempt. More often the writer falls into a happy ending and then retreats from it. Reynolds Price, for example, first chooses a triumphant ending for *A Whole New Life*: he states that his life since the discovery and treatment of a tumor in his spinal cord has been better than ever. But then he wonders what he is doing writing such a triumphant ending. "How self-deluding, self-serving, is that?" And continues: "Why do physically damaged people so often meet the world with clear bright eyes and what seem unjustified or lunatic smiles? Have some few layers of our minds burned off, leaving us dulled to the shocks of life, the actual state of our devastation?"⁶ While acknowledging the fact that being alive is itself worth celebrating, he still wonders if the celebration constitutes a retreat from acknowledgment of how difficult life with disability continues to be. "Are we merely displaying a normal animal pleasure in being at least alive and breathing, not outward bound to the dark unknown or anxious for some illusory safety, some guarantee we know to be ludicrous?"⁷

Price is right to question his own ending. Because his book in no way sugarcoats the suffering he endured, his statement that he is happier since his cancer rings false. The book itself describes a life torn apart by a brutal series of events: repeated surgeries, radiation, rehabilitation, and continued severe pain. While no doubt Price is telling the truth that he is happy in his present life, he himself knows that he must also acknowledge the terrible pain he has been through. By questioning his own ending he remains true to his book.

Lawrence Langer notices among Holocaust survivors a similar tendency when ending their stories to first back away from the implications of the devastating story they have told and in so doing betray the complexity of their situation. One survivor first concludes, "It makes you a much stronger human being to fight for the right of humanity," but then he reconsiders. Finally he says, instead, that the Holocaust left people fundamentally damaged: "Anyone who went through this kind of atrocity ends up not being the way you should be."⁸ Langer offers another example that indicates how strong is the impetus to end the story as a triumph. He discusses Martin Gilbert, who writes about Nazi atrocities "with a ruthless and unsettling resolve not to masquerade the worst, leaving the reader heavy-hearted and bereft."⁹ Langer found himself incredulous when Gilbert ended his book "with an array of sentiments that he contradicts on almost every other page of his own chronicle."¹⁰ In fact, in his final paragraph Gilbert lists the many ways people resisted the Nazis and says, "Simply to survive was a victory of the human spirit."¹¹ So stunned is Langer that Gilbert employed the "grammar of heroism and martyrdom" to end his book that he checks to see if he remembered accurately. In fact, Langer confirms, nothing in the book supports this notion of a triumph of the human spirit. It is a book about the devastation of the human spirit.

Sometimes a book whose story acknowledges the serious difficulties involved in a life with illness simply ends with a summary of lessons learned that sound more triumphant than the story. Robert Lipsyte takes the reader through the ups and downs of his own testicular cancer and his ex-wife's death from breast cancer. The narrative ends with the very moving image of his son weeping as he embraces his mother's body. Lipsyte then tacks on to his narrative a kind of self-help section called "Mediquette,"[12] which offers tips on how to deal with doctors, nurses, insurance companies, family, and friends. Given that Lipsyte's book is subtitled *Comfort and Advice for the Journey*, it is not surprising that he adopts the persona of a travel guide taking people through the country of illness he calls "Malady." However, this preoccupation with advice-giving, mildly distracting throughout the book, takes over in "Mediquette." There his focus shifts from his portrayal of how devastating illness is to his suggestion that, after all, it is manageable, if you follow certain steps. The tone of the section seems out of place after such a moving depiction of the profound emotional impact of illness on him and his family's life.

Sometimes writers, realizing they have fallen into a triumphant ending, add an afterward or epilogue to set the record straight. They inform the reader that, in fact, the sentiments with which they ended their book do not reflect the difficult suffering and continual challenge they face in their life. They explain their life was actually much messier than their ending suggests. It is interesting that these writers, who could, despite their reservations, have left their triumphant ending, are sufficiently bothered by its oversimplification to reassert how complex their experience with illness has been.

In an epilogue to *A Nearly Normal Life* Charles Mee adds a section describing the difficulties in his life after the book ended. His written memoir ends as he goes off to Harvard to begin what the reader surmises will be a full and satisfying life, a triumph over polio. It is an eloquent and insightful story in which Mee speaks honestly about his painful struggle, but emerges as someone who makes an excellent adjustment to his disability and finds consolation in a creative life. And so the story ends.

So why does Mee add this raw epilogue in which he reveals the darker side of his adult life? Mee seems to want to set the record straight by explaining that he continues to deal with the physical and emotional repercussions of polio. As a result of postpolio syndrome—a general weakening that often occurs thirty or forty years after polio—he is not as steady on his feet as when he left for college, he recounts. He is losing strength in his shoulder and hand. He goes on to say that all he accomplished in his recovery from polio—going from being in bed unable to move to walking on crutches, figuring out that in his life he would need to rely on his mind rather than his body and then pursuing a productive adult life—"was not the end of the story."[13] As he puts it, "One does not achieve grace and then live forever after on a serene, unchanging glide path of bliss. Life continues to change. New things surface; old wounds hidden by bigger wounds show up when the bigger wounds are healed."[14]

Mee lays bare how difficult and unglamorous his emotional adjustment has been. "Physical damage is easy to repair; the psychic takes longer,"[15] he comments. For him "it also took years of heavy drinking, some drugs, a fall into a very deep depression, the love of more than one woman, three failed marriages"[16] before he begins writing plays. This epilogue functions as a kind of second ending to the book and one that leaves the reader with a very different feeling. Polio is not an event that Mee experienced in the past that can be neatly summed up in a triumphant ending. Rather, it is a disease that continues to have an impact on his body and psyche. By providing a more complicated ending, Mee deprives readers of the chance to move on from the story as if all is settled. Instead he insists we understand the complexity of life after polio.

In completing my own memoir about breast cancer, I went through a similar process of rewriting the ending. I conclude the actual narrative with a conversation I had with my daughter, Molly, who was seven at the time. She asks, "'Is it over, Mom?' I ask, 'Is what over, honey?' 'Breast cancer,' she replies. 'Yes, Molly,' I answer, 'Breast cancer is over.'"[17] The reader knows from what I had said earlier in my story that I have no idea if cancer is over, and in fact, am terrified that it may not be. I offer the happy ending because I feel Molly needs it, and perhaps I and the reader need it, but at best it is a wish. This ending is an attempt to suggest that I am aware that I do not know if my cancer is over, but for the moment I choose to believe it is.

I wrote and eventually discarded an afterword in which I abandoned the complexity of that ending and catalogued the lessons I learned from breast cancer. Upon reflection I realized that I had written a triumphant ending that in no way fit a book in which I concluded that I had found the experience "without redeeming value." But I also realized how powerful was my own wish to wrap up the story neatly and to sound like a wise person who had learned something from the experience. I then wrote a new afterword in which I described the rejected afterword as an expression of my wish to leave my children a more triumphant narrative with a more likeable, heroic mother. I ended the new afterword by describing a fantasy of the mother of Victorian literature who lay dying in her bed in an upstairs bedroom surrounded by her family. My intention this time was to suggest more explicitly the unknown and not necessarily triumphant nature of the woman's experience. "In my fantasy, the mother faces death calmly in the comfort of that love. Or does she?" I then go on to say, "I've always wondered what it was actually like for the woman in the bed. Was anyone really with her in her dying? Did she feel held in her family's love or totally alone, isolated in her own closed circle?"[18]

Sometimes a happy ending, while understandable when an outcome is good, may ring false to the reader as the ending of an illness story. The journalist Joyce Wadler wrote *My Breast* about her diagnosis and treatment for breast cancer. The author's account of her journey from the shock of diagnosis through the ups and downs of treatment is serious and engaging. Her ending, however, an upbeat fantasy about her future, seems too much of a departure from the seriousness of her experience. She imagines lying in bed with a future boyfriend who asks about the scar on her breast and she responds, "Glad you asked, 'cause it's a *wonderful* story."[19] By calling it a wonderful story Wadler goes beyond even the typical triumphant ending and abandons the tone of the book itself.

This was Wadler's first cancer. Given a relatively good prognosis, she had reason to be optimistic. At the age of forty-seven, however, four years after her breast cancer, Wadler was diagnosed with third-stage ovarian cancer. She then wrote a two-part article for *New York Magazine* much in the sassy, clever style of *My Breast* but with a more somber and chastened tone.[20] She underwent a fairly brutal regime of treatments—two surgeries, chemotherapy, and interperitoneal therapy (chemo delivered directly to the abdomen).

Shaken by this experience, she looks back on her breast cancer experience and describes how smug she felt then as opposed to now. "I know just two things about ovarian cancer. It's vicious, and it killed Gilda Radner."[21] She refers to her first cancer as her "big career break, when cancer was amusing."[22] But things are different with ovarian cancer. "The cancer has not all been removed—it is worse than the sonogram indicated, and it has spread."[23] She has trouble regaining her confidence this time. "And now I just can't seem to get back on the horse, or whatever the expression is."[24] Wadler ends this first installment with a description of herself joking with friends, but this time the content is far more serious than the fantasy with which she ends *My Breast.* In the midst of this joking she remembers the part in the novel *The World According to Garp* "'where the gunner who got shot can only say his name—Garp—and then he gets worse and he can't remember the *G* and he can only say "Arp," and then he loses the *p*? That's what's happening to me.'"[25] She leaves the reader with this quite sobering image of the gunner who is left, as the result of damage to his brain, with holes in his identity. It represents the many and continued losses in her life. Wadler's two different stories of cancer demonstrate how the seriousness of a person's illness sometimes determines how much an awareness of mortality enters into the end of the narrative.

As I explained in the preceding chapter, Donald Hall intended *Life Work* to be about the daily routine of a writer's life but ended up writing about a writer's life interrupted by a recurrence of colon cancer. He ends the first half of his book with his diagnosis, a description of his grief at the possibility of dying and of his realization that he is writing in defiance of death. The second half is essentially a meditation on the question of writing as a way to transcend mortality. His acute awareness of the possibility of death changes the nature of the work. For example, rather than imagine possible writing projects for the future, he wonders how lethargy and nausea will affect his plans. Should he cut short the long poem he's been writing for fifteen years—"do I need to rewrite the other third or merely cut it out, like the lobe of a liver?"[26] This metaphor of a diseased liver recurs throughout and reminds us that the cancer will determine how long his life and work will continue. What is striking is that he maintains the tone of the earlier part of the book—meandering, musing about plans, while also communicating the very different ways he thinks about his continuing work. Now he knows that his work is contingent on his continued health. He informs the reader of how his awareness of death affects him at every turn. While writing cannot obliterate the reality of his cancer, it can absorb him even as he lives with the awareness of his illness and of the fact that death will have the final word. "This book ends otherwise than it started."[27]

The end of John Diamond's *Cowards Get Cancer Too* reflects the dilemma of a writer whose disease is serious enough to kill him. Diamond does not know whether his tongue cancer has been eradicated or not. He recognizes that "there's every chance that by the time this appears in the bookshops it [cancer] will all be over"[28] with only some lingering damage and some scars. But he has a hunch that the cancer will return. He ends his story with a summing up of what he has learned, but then pulls back and acknowledges these are lessons he could have learned without cancer. Ultimately, his ending reveals his true feelings, including a kind of bitterness: "But the bad has outweighed the good a millionfold. . . . It shouldn't be like this. That I can face the fact that it is like this is, I suppose, something. But what a bloody meager something it is."[29] This is a rather shocking statement coming after what was some attempt to reach some kind of positive ending.

Diamond held off writing an afterword in the hope that he would be able to say "something less equivocating" about whether he would live or die. When he finally does end the book, he still can't write anything certain. While his biopsies are clear he is not convinced he is all right. When he learned of his cancer a year earlier he had promised his wife that he would not commit suicide, he says; now he wonders if he would have made that promise had he known what the year would be like. He has lost weight; his speech is halting; he has scars, constant pain in his throat and an associated earache; he needs to sit up when he sleeps because his lack of saliva glands causes mucous problems; he has no taste, and he experiences coughing fits, anger, depression, and tiredness that he fears may indicate recurrent cancer. He goes on to tell the reader he appreciates his wife and children more and he doesn't apologize for cancer making that the reason. He ends with this statement: "I still don't believe that there is any sense in which the cancer has been a good thing, but, well, it is strange, isn't it?"[30]

When the book was reprinted in paperback the afterword was followed with a postscript Diamond wrote to fill the reader in on what happened to him in the intervening months. He had the rest of his tongue removed, but still the cancer returned. He explains that, before another planned surgery, this time to remove his voice box, he faces what he calls "the prospect of the tongueless, voiceless, foodless life." His doctors take him into a comfortable room to give him the bad news that there is too much cancer for surgery to be effective; he might have six months to live, maybe longer with chemo. He ends this postscript by talking about his realization that he needs to make plans, to tell the kids, and to celebrate his anniversary with his wife. Much as he did in ending his afterword, Diamond calls it strange: "It's strange, isn't it, how in the middle of all this madness there are some things worth celebrating?"[31] He draws the analogy to any forty-five-year-old who goes about his business aware but not always attending to the fact of his mortality. That forty-five-year-old doesn't say, "Why bother going to the movies? I'll be dead in fifty years." He, likewise, goes about getting a dog because "a dog is a happy thing, and it will be happy for me for whatever time I've got left and as happy as things can be for the family when I've gone."[32]

It's difficult to know what to make of Diamond's multiple endings. He has been criticized for writing a book that feels thrown together. Since Diamond's prognosis is ever-changing and increasingly grim, the narrative inevitably has a disrupted and unsettled quality. But there remains the question of how one tells such an unsettling story. Should the book itself feel messy and unsettled, thereby suggesting what it is really like to be dealing with a devastating cancer? Or should the writer provide us with some sense of resolution even when there really is none? Or is there something in the middle—a story that tells the truth about the devastating experience of cancer but is presented in a way we can handle?

Often the difficulty ending an illness narrative reflects the fact that one needs to bring narrative closure when in fact the future of one's health remains an open question. As I finished my book, *Ordinary Life*, I was faced with a decision about whether to include information about new health problems that had arisen for me. The week the proofs of my book arrived I was diagnosed with a new cancer of the lymph system whose exact diagnosis was still a subject of debate among pathologists. (It turned out to be Hodgkin's disease). I struggled with whether to change the book's ending to include this information or to end the book as it was written. Realizing that a memoir must stop at some point in the story of a life, and also that the story had a certain integrity that might be disrupted by a change, I decided not to mention the new diagnosis and I left the story as written—that despite worries about the future I had essentially returned to ordinary life. I realize now that I could have included the information about a new cancer and that such an ending would have mirrored the fact that the outcome of that cancer was unknown. In a sense I opted for the resolution provided by a happier ending, perhaps finding the other possibility—telling how my future had become more precarious—too difficult to admit or too unresolved as an ending.

The question of the ending of life and a life story is at the center of Julian Barnes's commentary on the ending of Daudet's notes. Barnes tells us that it is not clear when Daudet stopped writing his notes. Although it is believed he stopped three years before he died, Barnes points out that one note, in fact, refers to a visit to Venice that happened only eighteen months before his death. Because the notes come to no real conclusion but break off rather abruptly, our curiosity is aroused about why they end when they do. Barnes offers various possibilities. He quotes Andre Ebner, who offers one theory: that Daudet's passion for his work—reading and discussing ideas—was stronger than his illness, and that he stopped examining his illness because he chose instead to talk with other patients, thus transforming "his unceasing torments into a goodness which increased with each day."[33] While Barnes offers evidence that supports Ebner's notion that Daudet was a compassionate and generous man who entertained the other patients at the thermal spa with his reading, lively talk, and wisdom—he then offers another point of view. According to Daudet's son Leon, his father never gave up examining his illness and would not have been likely to give up his own writing. Leon paraphrases Daudet: "There are a great many different kinds of instruments belonging to the executioner; if they do not scare you too much, examine them carefully. It is with our torments as it is with shadows. Attention clears them up and drives them away."[34] We are left not really knowing if Daudet stopped the notes where he did because he had solved his literary problem, lost interest in the subject, become more involved with other people who were ill, or was simply too sick to write.

Barnes points out that Daudet lived with a terrible fear of "total paralysis, aphasia and imbecility."[35] According to Leon, Daudet was spared the terrible death he had feared: Daudet collapsed and died during a pleasant dinner with his family. But Barnes argues that Leon's recollection of his father's death is too pat and a bit romanticized. "As an ending this is neat, and a little novelistic."[36] He points out that, according to the medical reports, two doctors came and spent an hour and a half trying to revive Daudet, first by giving him artificial respiration by a then popular but gruesome technique of pulling on the tongue and then by attempting to stimulate the diaphragm. To his credit, the account Barnes offers of Daudet's last months keeps open the question of Daudet's last days. Those around Daudet wanted to romanticize his story in a way not necessarily in keeping with Daudet's unflinching and clear-eyed view of illness and death. Barnes challenges each of them. When Ebner depicts a saint-like Daudet abruptly giving up his contemplation of illness, Barnes offers evidence to the contrary. When Leon describes his father's actual death as peaceful, Barnes offers details of a more complicated death.

The attention Barnes pays in this edition to the ending of Daudet's notes and the end of his life serves as a reminder that the interests of truth and the interests of narrative often come into conflict at a person's death. When someone dies it takes little time for people to begin composing their version of the deceased person's life and death, usually a mix of fact and fiction. In Daudet's case what remains true is that we know very little about the time close to his death. Just as his disjointed notes prove a good form for representing the disrupted nature of illness, this ending clouded in mystery fits the story of his illness and dying.

The ending of Daudet's notes, because they break off abruptly, leaves us with a sense of the author's departure. Sometimes choice of language suggests a similar kind of winding down of life. Abba Kovner, the poet who had been a leader of the Jewish resistance in the Vilna ghetto, wrote a collection of poems entitled "Sloan Kettering" in which he chronicled his experience with the cancer that led to his death. After his vocal cords were removed he could no longer speak. He wrote short verses that were spare and direct. He writes that he "cannot exist / without meaning / without probing to the end / of this sudden muteness" and then suggests "perhaps absence of speech/ also has meaning."[37] The reviewer Edward Hirsch described this poetry as "an art pared away to what is absolutely essential, an art of making language at the edge of a void where everything is undone, unmade."[38] One senses in Kovner's poetry his departure from the work, his move into silence. This is both the content and form of his poetry.

Sometimes things happen after a book is completed and the protagonist has died that the author feels should be included as part of the story. Of course this is only possible in a narrative written by someone other than the ill person. The first page of Fenton Johnson's book *Geography of the Heart*, about his lover's dying of AIDS, simply says "Prologue/Postscript," a heading that indicates the nonlinear dimension of this story.[39] In it Johnson describes a visit to his lover's parents after their son has died. This prologue to the book is actually the postscript to his lover's death; that is, it happened after the narrative of his lover's dying. This framing of the story underlines the fact that whereas the writer's lover dies, that death is part of the ongoing life of his parents and his lover. By structuring the book this way Johnson suggests that death is part of everyone's life.

When those of us who write about illness and disability come to the end of our story, we find ourselves in quite a tangle. On the one hand, we are writing a story and we have the sense that a story calls for closure. On the other hand, we are writing about illness and mortality, our own mortality, and however good a story we tell, the fact of our mortality inevitably complicates the ending. While a happy ending may work for an acute illness, it simply doesn't work for a chronic one or an illness whose outcome is unknown. In these situations the nature of illness poses serious problems for the writing of the story and results in all kinds of endings—confused, appropriately open-ended, ironic, eloquent about the complexity of life.

And yet these problematic endings are perhaps most fitting for an illness story. There is a wonderful section of Hall's book that illustrates the limits of writing in the face of death. Hall is observing the way writing and the life of the imagination allow him to transcend his cancer. He explains that in his own experience writing can give him the sense of uninterrupted time separate from illness. He then recalls a clever quatrain Stanley Kunitz wrote when he was twenty about his father, who died before Kunitz was born. It reads:

Observe the wisdom of the Florentine
Who, feeling death upon him, scribbled fast
To make revision, of a deathbed scene,
Gloating that he was accurate at last.[40]

Hall reads these lines as suggesting that death is a stimulus to work. I read them as representing the irony faced by all writers. The poet continues to write even as death threatens to end his work and life, gloating that he knows the resolution at last. Absorbed in his success, he pays little heed to what the reader and the poet who describes the Florentine know—that he has no control over his real deathbed scene or over the time or manner of his death. Art will not allow him to transcend death.

Or will it? The poet's writing did in fact absorb him in an uninterrupted flow of thought and enable him to go on doing what he loved in life. Perhaps the apparently self-deceiving poet is wiser than he seems.

Conclusion

In the history of art the late works are the catastrophes.
—Theodor Adorno, quoted by Edward Said, *On Late Style*

In his later years Edward Said, the writer and critic, living with his own diagnosis of cancer, became interested in the style of great writers and musicians at the end of their lives. Said acknowledged that certain artistic works live up to our "accepted notion of age and wisdom" in that they reflect "a special maturity, a new spirit of reconciliation and serenity often expressed in terms of a miraculous transfiguration of common reality."[1] Yet he was fascinated by Theodor Adorno's analysis of Beethoven's late works–his Ninth Symphony, for example, as characterized not by "harmony and resolution" but by "intransigence, difficulty and unresolved contradiction."[2] Some people have a more conflicted or even tortured experience in the face of the body's decay and approaching death, Said suggests, and their art may reflect, rather than transcend, the complexity of that experience. For Said, as for Adorno, the late compositions of some artists reflect not a sense of resolution but of "'lost totality,' and are therefore catastrophic."[3]

The writers I discuss in this book attempt to describe the "lost totality," the "catastrophes" they have experienced in their lives as a result of illness or accident. Generally, we think of writing about illness as an attempt to impose order on experiences that are chaotic. But it becomes apparent in reading these memoirs that certain writers are equally interested in representing in words the irreconcilable, fragmented, interrupted, or even chaotic nature of their experience. They do not necessarily succeed in creating a work that in itself is an embodiment of what is irreconcilable, as Said believes Beethoven was able to do. But they do show us that damage done by illness or accident is not easily transcended by a resilient self; rather, damage compromises the very self needed for transcendence. They also demonstrate how hard it is to represent in words or form what is so painful in their experience. Their attempts to do so, even their frustrated attempts, indicate both the challenge that is illness and the limits of language and storytelling in the face of it.

Given how difficult living with illness or disability can be, it is striking that the triumph narrative continues to hold such sway in our culture. Most of us harbor the fear that we might not be very brave in the face of serious illness; even a suspicious blood test result or the need for further x-rays terrifies us with the possibility that we are about to be propelled into the dreaded world of illness. We have seen pain and depression and dying among our loved ones and know how soul-sapping these experiences can be. And yet we live with this cultural story of triumph that suggests any adversity can be managed or overcome.

Those who offer the different story that serious illness is overwhelming, even devastating, are seen to be doing something daring. Reviewers describe them as "unflinching," "candid," "brutally honest," or "courageous" with the suggestion that it takes daring to acknowledge the painful and unmanageable aspects of illness. And yet, I would argue, these stories are not sensational or frightening as those adjectives suggest, but comforting in their honesty about experiences with which we are all familiar. They describe the pain, frustration, despair, humor, and love that constitute life. Here are people who, in the face of devastating experience, try to keep on living and reflect on even the most difficult aspects of their life. In doing so they suggest that one can be ill without adopting the attitudes of a mystic or the bravery of a soldier.

It is too soon to know whether these stories are part of a cultural shift away from the narrative of triumph or whether they represent an ongoing but less dominant strand in writing about illness. Although most of these books were written during the past three decades, fewer such books have appeared of late. Joan Didion's *The Year of Magical Thinking* is an exception. Didion's book quickly appeared on the best-seller list in 2005 and received high praise from critics. Readers came to know the dimensions of Didion's grief over her husband's death and daughter's illness. They also became part of a kind of community of people talking with each other about Didion's book and, consequently, about illness and death.

Authors who venture to tell a story that includes what is disruptive and even overwhelming are joining with others in society who see a need to acknowledge what is devastating about illness and disability. There are American journalists writing about veterans of the Iraq war who are struggling to live with severe disabilities. A global movement to ameliorate suffering from AIDS reflects an awareness of the extent of suffering from this disease. Critics of our health care system recognize that poorly organized and delivered care can in itself be a source of suffering.

Acknowledgment of the reality of serious illness and disability and what they entail can foster an understanding of the difficult issues people face. With such understanding, perhaps those who wish to decline high-tech treatments when there is little chance for cure will not be met with an insistence that they continue to fight. Perhaps people who live with chronic illness or the possibility of recurrence can feel they are not alone in a world of people who have triumphed. Perhaps those of us who visit our dying friends might feel able to forgo hollow platitudes about recovery and admit that we are at a loss for words.

Different societal reactions also become possible when we acknowledge the reality of suffering and our human limitations in the face of it. Doctors and patients alike might be more willing to admit when cure is not possible. If we acknowledge that not all disease can be cured we might provide adequately for hospice and palliative care services. If we face that the treatment for AIDS is not simply a triumph but involves a life on chemotherapy, we might design better educational and prevention programs. If we understand the randomness of illness and accident, we might stop blaming the ill for their suffering and stop relegating them to a world distant from ours.

Unflinching stories about illness and injury are not easy to embrace. Not everyone can or will embrace them, and most of us have little idea how we would frame or live out our own serious illness. The important thing is that these stories of illness as unmanageable and even devastating are available alongside other stories. If they resonate with our experience, they may give us a sense that we are not alone. They may also show us that facing rather than denying the complex nature of serious illness can be liberating, the beginning of dealing with it.

Susan Sontag's response a few years ago to her diagnosis of myelodysplastic syndrome, a virulent blood cancer, points out the complexity inherent in anyone's choice about how to respond to serious illness. After years of repudiating the widespread use of the battle metaphor for illness, Sontag spent the final months before she died battling with all her resources against her third cancer. Sontag's point was never to deny those who are ill the right to fight the forces of disease, but rather, to insist that the metaphor of battle, particularly in regard to cancer, could have negative repercussions for the person who is ill. In an attempt to triumph over her own cancer she spared no expense and no pain for herself as she pursued radical and experimental treatments. But she did so without illusions about illness and knowing full well what she was taking on. Her son David Rieff describes the torturous treatments she was willing to undergo even with a slim chance of survival. "There are those who can reconcile themselves to death and those who can't,"[4] he comments. Sontag chose not to reconcile herself.

What is significant is that Sontag had a choice. Because she and others were willing to insist that no one has a right to tell another how to cope with or view illness, she had a choice about whether to approach her illness as a battle or not. By applying all her intellectual acumen to the task of uncovering the coercive effect of language about fighting illness, she made it possible to decline the battle. And yet, when her moment came, she chose to struggle to the end.

Why is the discussion of language and narrative form so relevant to our understanding of serious illness and disability? People write to stay alive, to communicate their experience to others, and achieve a measure of immortality, but the reality of illness and the body point to the ultimate limits on our ability to transcend illness and dying through writing. Attempting to put the experience of serious illness and disability into words is like life itself: it is about confronting limits, acknowledging chaos, and, within that chaos, trying to make sense of what is happening. Illness and disability are in their essence a confrontation with limits. Some writers eschew coercive formulae for dealing with pain or diminished bodily function and the consequent feelings of loss and helplessness. Instead they describe the landscape of desolation and brokenness that illness and disability create. Within that landscape they and their readers can contemplate whether and how, beyond literature, they can speak in the face of wordlessness, remain whole in the face of brokenness, and find meaning and consolation in the face of death.

— Notes —

Introduction

1. Reynolds Price, *A Whole New Life* (New York: Scribners Classics, 1994), 180.
2. Kathlyn Conway, *Ordinary Life: A Memoir of Illness* (New York: W. H. Freeman), 1997.
3. Price, *A Whole New Life*, 180.
4. Nancy Mairs, in Foreword to G. Thomas Couser, *Recovering Bodies: Illness, Disability, and Life Writing* (Madison: University of Wisconsin Press, 1997), x.
5. Arthur W. Frank, *The Wounded Storyteller: Body, Illness, & Ethics* (Chicago: University of Chicago Press, 1995), 77.
6. Frank, *The Wounded Storyteller*, 79–80.
7. G. Thomas Couser, *Recovering Bodies: Illness, Disability, and Life Writing* (Madison: University of Wisconsin Press, 1997), 5.
8. Couser, *Recovering Bodies*, 39.
9. Norman Cousins, *Anatomy of an Illness as Perceived by the Patient: Reflections on Healing and Regeneration* (New York: Norton, 1979); Bernie Siegel, *Love, Medicine and Miracles: Lessons Learned about Self-Healing from a Surgeon's Experience with Exceptional Patients* (New York: Harper and Row, 1986); Andrew Weil, *Spontaneous Healing: How to Discover and Enhance Your Body's Ability to Maintain and Heal Itself* (New York: Alfred A. Knopf, 1995); Deepak Chopra, *Creating Health: How to Wake Up the Body's Intelligence* (Boston: Houghton Mifflin, 1991).
10. Chopra, *Creating Health*, 69.
11. Chopra, *Creating Health*, 70–71.
12. Weil, *Spontaneous Healing*, 23.
13. Esther Sternberg, *The Balance Within: The Science Connecting Health and Emotions* (New York: W. H. Freeman, 2000).
14. The March 15, 2004, issue of *Cancer* reports on an Australian study that concludes that "patients with a positive attitude fared no better than their less upbeat peers."
15. Christina Middlebrook, *Seeing the Crab: A Memoir of Dying Before I Do* (New York: Doubleday, 1996), 4.

16. Middlebrook, *Seeing the Crab,* 4.

17. Heather Jose, *Letters to Sydney: Hope, Faith and Cancer* (Bloomington, Ind.: Authorhouse, 2004), 160.

18. John Gunther, *Death Be Not Proud: A Memoir* (New York: Harper Perennial, 1949).

19. Betty Rollins, *First You Cry* (New York: HarperCollins, 1976).

20. Lance Armstrong with Sally Jenkins, *It's Not About the Bike: My Journey Back to Life* (New York: Berkley Books, 2000).

21. Elisabeth Kübler-Ross, *On Death and Dying* (New York: Touchstone, 1969).

22. Susan Sontag, *Illness as Metaphor and AIDS and Its Metaphors* (New York: Anchor, 1989).

23. Sherwin B. Nuland, *How We Die: Reflections on Life's Final Chapter* (New York: Vintage Books, 1995).

24. Arlene Croce, "Discussing the Undiscussable," *New Yorker,* December 26, 1994, 54.

25. Richard Goldstein, "The Croce Criterion," *Village Voice,* January 3, 1995, 8.

26. Patrick Smith, "What Memory Forgets," *The Nation,* July 27–August 3, 1998, 30.

27. Smith, "What Memory Forgets," 30.

28. Laura Miller, "The Last Word," *New York Times Book Review,* February 8, 2004, 31.

29. Morris Dickstein, *New York Times Book Review,* February 9, 2003, 10.

30. Virginia Woolf, *On Being Ill* (Ashfield, Mass.: Paris Press, 2002).

31. James Fenton, "Turgenev's Banana," *New York Review of Books,* February 13, 2003.

32. Julian Barnes, introduction to Alphonse Daudet, *In the Land of Pain,* trans. by Julian Barnes (New York: Alfred A. Knopf, 2002).

33. Leonard Kriegel, "The Body of Imagination," *The Nation,* November 9, 1998, 26.

34. Joan Didion, *The Year of Magical Thinking* (New York: Alfred A. Knopf, 2005).

35. Arthur Kleinman, *The Illness Narratives: Suffering, Healing and the Human Condition* (New York: Basic Books, 1998), xii.

36. Kathryn Montgomery Hunter, *Doctors' Stories: The Narrative Structure of Medical Knowledge* (Princeton: Princeton University Press, 1991).

37. Anne Hunsaker Hawkins, *Reconstructing Illness: Studies in Pathography* (West Lafayette, Ind.: Purdue University Press, 1993).

38. Hunter argues that "only recently, as we have begun to live long enough to fall victim to chronic disease, have very many stories been written to examine illness as the individual experiences it" (*Doctors' Stories,* 153). Hawkins states, "As a genre, pathography is remarkable in that it seems to

have emerged *ex nihilo;* book-length personal accounts of illness are uncommon before 1950 and rarely found before 1900" (*Reconstructing Illness*, 3). Couser suggests (in his introduction) that the proliferation of illness narrators may mirror the tendency of marginal groups after the civil rights movement to assert their right to speak. Leonard Kriegel cites a greater number of books that deal with the actual bodily experience of illness and its ramifications. He observes, "In essays, memoirs, poems and plays, if rarely in fiction, the ills to which flesh is heir are now examined without sentimentality" ("The Body of Imagination," 26). Earlier writing about illness was generally found in private correspondence or religious tracts or sermons, not in the form of a personal narrative.

39. Daudet, *In the Land of Pain;* Woolf, *On Being Ill.*

40. Anatole Broyard, *Intoxicated by My Illness and Other Writings on Life and Death* (New York: Fawcett Columbine, 1992), 20.

41. Harold Brodkey, *This Wild Darkness: The Story of My Death* (New York: Metropolitan, 1996) 172–73.

42. Robert Murphy, *The Body Silent: The Different World of the Disabled* (New York: Norton, 1990), 29.

Chapter 1

1. Middlebrook, *Seeing the Crab*, 114.

2. Marjorie Williams, *The Woman at the Washington Zoo: Writings on Politics, Family and Fate* (New York: Public Affairs, 2005), 335.

3. Williams, *Woman at Washington Zoo*, 335.

4. Margaret Edson, *Wit* (New York: Faber and Faber, 1993), 5.

5. *Webster's Third New International Dictionary* (Springfield, Mass.: G. and C. Merriam Company, 1961), 1497.

6. Hawkins, *Reconstructing Illness.*

7. Barbara Ehrenreich, "Welcome to Cancerland: A Mammogram Leads to a Cult of Pink Kitsch," *Harper's*, November 2001, 50.

8. Richard Seltzer, *Raising the Dead: A Doctor's Encounter with His Own Mortality* (New York: Viking, 1993).

9. Seltzer, *Raising the Dead*, 112.

10. Brodkey, *This Wild Darkness*, 46–47.

11. Mark Doty, *Heaven's Coast: A Memoir* (New York: HarperCollins, 1996), 157.

12. Williams, *Woman at Washington Zoo*, 335.

13. Andrew Solomon, *The Noonday Demon: An Atlas of Depression* (New York: Scribner, 2001), 135.

14. Christopher Reeve, *Still Me* (New York: Random House, 1998), 111.

15. Charles Mee, *A Nearly Normal Life* (New York: Little, Brown, 1999).

16. Mee, *A Nearly Normal Life*, 61.

17. Mee, *A Nearly Normal Life*, 58.

18. Mee, *A Nearly Normal Life*, 60.
19. Mee, *A Nearly Normal Life*, 59.
20. Mee, *A Nearly Normal Life*, 37–38.
21. Mee, *A Nearly Normal Life*, 40.
22. Mee, *A Nearly Normal Life*, 175.
23. Mee, *A Nearly Normal Life*, 87.
24. Mee, *A Nearly Normal Life*, 82.
25. Mee, *A Nearly Normal Life*, 83.
26. Mee, *A Nearly Normal Life*, 91.
27. Mee, *A Nearly Normal Life*, 92.
28. Mee, *A Nearly Normal Life*, 92.
29. Mee, *A Nearly Normal Life*, 93.
30. Mee, *A Nearly Normal Life*, 92–93.
31. Leonard Kriegel, *Falling into Life* (San Francisco: North Point Press, 1991).
32. Kriegel, *Falling into Life*, 11.
33. Kriegel, *Falling into Life*, 55–60.
34. Stephen Kuusisto, *Planet of the Blind: A Memoir* (New York: Dial Press, 1998).
35. Kriegel, *Falling into Life*, 60.
36. Kriegel, *Falling into Life*, 132.
37. Kriegel, *Falling into Life*, 64.
38. Kriegel, *Falling into Life*, 65.
39. Kriegel, *Falling into Life*, 66.
40. Kriegel, *Falling into Life*, 152.
41. Kriegel, *Falling into Life*, 155.
42. Kriegel, *Falling into Life*, 155.
43. Kriegel, *Falling into Life*, 155.
44. Kuusisto, *Planet of the Blind*, 41.
45. Kuusisto, *Planet of the Blind*, 99.
46. Kuusisto, *Planet of the Blind*, 132.
47. Kuusisto, *Planet of the Blind*, 132.
48. Georgina Kleege, *Sight Unseen* (New Haven: Yale University Press, 1999).
49. Kleege, *Sight Unseen*, 16.
50. Oliver Sacks, *A Leg to Stand On* (New York: Harper Perennial, 1993).
51. Sacks, *Leg to Stand On*, 69.
52. Sacks, *Leg to Stand On*, 70.
53. Sacks, *Leg to Stand On*, 80.
54. Sacks, *Leg to Stand On*, 81.
55. Sacks, *Leg to Stand On*, 82.
56. Sacks, *Leg to Stand On*, 83.
57. Sacks, *Leg to Stand On*, 84.
58. Solomon, *The Noonday Demon*, 84.

59. Solomon, *The Noonday Demon*, 84.
60. Mairs, *Waist-High*, 6.
61. Mairs, *Waist-High*, 125.
62. Mairs, *Waist-High*, 126.
63. Mairs, *Waist-High*, 126.
64. Frank, *The Wounded Storyteller*, 3.
65. Kleinman, *The Illness Narratives*, xi–xii.

Chapter 2

1. Solomon, *The Noonday Demon*, 49–50.
2. Robert Lipsyte, *In the Country of Illness: Comfort and Advice for the Journey* (New York: Alfred A. Knopf, 1998), 115–16.
3. Max Lerner, *Wrestling with the Angel: A Memoir of My Triumph over Illness* (New York: Norton, 1990), 24.
4. Murphy, *The Body Silent*, 12.
5. Brodkey, *This Wild Darkness*, 173.
6. Price, *A Whole New Life*, 179.
7. Nancy Smith, "'To Return, to Eat, to Tell the Story': Primo Levi's Lessons on Living and Dying in the Aftermath of Trauma," *International Forum of Psychoanalysis* 13, nos. 1–2 (2004): 66–69.
8. Levi quoted by Smith, "To Return," 66–67.
9. Levi quoted by Smith, "To Return," 67.
10. Susanna Kaysen, *Girl Interrupted* (New York: Vintage, 1993).
11. Murphy in *The Body Silent* uses the designations "damaged self" and "disembodied self."
12. Murphy, *The Body Silent*, 108.
13. Robert McCrum, *My Year Off* (New York: Broadway Books, 1998).
14. McCrum, *My Year Off*, 73.
15. McCrum, *My Year Off*, 172.
16. Lucy Grealy, *Autobiography of a Face* (New York: Houghton Mifflin, 1994).
17. McCrum, *My Year Off*, 13.
18. McCrum, *My Year Off*, 153.
19. Sacks, *Leg to Stand On*, 46.
20. Sacks, *Leg to Stand On*, 51.
21. Sacks, *Leg to Stand On*, 54.
22. Sacks, *Leg to Stand On*, 50.
23. Mairs, *Waist-High*, 43.
24. Mairs, *Waist-High*, 8–9.
25. Mairs, *Waist-High*, 9.
26. Floyd Skloot, *The Night-Side: Chronic Fatigue Syndrome and the Illness Experience* (Brownsville, Oreg.: Story Line Press, 1996).
27. Skloot, *The Night-Side*, 3.

28. Skloot, *The Night-Side*, 3–4.
29. Skloot, *The Night-Side*, 6.
30. Skloot, *The Night-Side*, 4.
31. Laura Hillenbrand, "A Sudden Illness—How My Life Changed," *New Yorker*, July 7, 2003, 58.
32. Ehrenreich, "Welcome to Cancerland," 44.
33. Ehrenreich, "Welcome to Cancerland," 44.
34. Ehrenreich, "Welcome to Cancerland," 45.
35. Ehrenreich, "Welcome to Cancerland," 45.
36. Ehrenreich, "Welcome to Cancerland," 45.
37. Murphy, *The Body Silent*, 100.
38. Murphy, *The Body Silent*, 100.
39. Murphy, *The Body Silent*, 101.
40. Murphy, *The Body Silent*, 101.
41. Middlebrook, *Seeing the Crab*, 55–56.
42. Middlebrook, *Seeing the Crab*, 56.
43. Middlebrook, *Seeing the Crab*, 56.
44. Grealy, *Autobiography of a Face*, 157.
45. Middlebrook, *Seeing the Crab*, 62.
46. Middlebrook, *Seeing the Crab*, 63.
47. Middlebrook, *Seeing the Crab*, 62.
48. John M. Hull, *Touching the Rock: An Experience of Blindness* (New York: Pantheon, 1990).
49. Hull, *Touching the Rock*, 152.
50. Hull, *Touching the Rock*, 153.
51. Stewart Alsop, *Stay of Execution: A Sort of Memoir* (New York: J. B. Lippincott, 1973), 20.
52. Alsop, *Stay of Execution*, 20.
53. Alsop, *Stay of Execution*, 21.
54. Alsop, *Stay of Execution*, 20.
55. Brodkey, *This Wild Darkness*, 67.
56. Lerner, *Wrestling with the Angel*, 28.

Chapter 3

1. Jean-Dominique Bauby, *The Diving Bell and the Butterfly* (New York: Alfred A. Knopf, 1997), 3.
2. John Diamond, *Because Cowards Get Cancer Too: A Hypochondriac Confronts His Nemesis* (New York: Random House, 1998) 118.
3. Randy Shilts, *And the Band Played On: Politics, People and the AIDs Epidemic* (New York: St. Martin's Press, 1987), 12.
4. Hawkins, *Reconstructing Illness*, 15. Hawkins refers in this regard to a number of theorists: Richard Olney's *Metaphors of Self*, Michael Sprinker's

Fictions of the Self, John Morris's *Versions of the Self,* Patricia Meyer Spacks's *Imaging a Self,* and John O. Lyons's *The Invention of the Self.*

5. Kriegel, *Falling into Life,* 41.
6. Kriegel, *Falling into Life,* 53.
7. Kriegel, *Falling into Life,* 89.
8. Kriegel, *Falling into Life,* 54.
9. Kriegel, *Falling into Life,* 44.
10. Reeve, *Still Me,* 5.
11. Reeve, *Still Me,* 278.
12. Reeve, *Still Me,* 274.
13. Price, *A Whole New Life,* 183.
14. Price, *A Whole New Life,* 183.
15. Price, *A Whole New Life,* 184.
16. Price, *A Whole New Life,* 188.
17. Price, *A Whole New Life,* 184.
18. Price, *A Whole New Life,* 189.
19. Audre Lorde, *The Cancer Journals* (San Francisco: Aunt Lute, 1980), 16.
20. Lorde, *The Cancer Journals,* 42.
21. Lorde, *The Cancer Journals,* 57.
22. Lorde, *The Cancer Journals,* 59.
23. Lorde, *The Cancer Journals,* 59.
24. Lorde, *The Cancer Journals,* 59.
25. Kay Redfield Jamison, *An Unquiet Mind: A Memoir of Moods and Madness* (New York: Vintage, 1996), 120.
26. Jamison, *An Unquiet Mind,* 120.
27. Jamison, *An Unquiet Mind,* 121.
28. Jamison, *An Unquiet Mind,* 121.
29. McCrum, *My Year Off,* 173.
30. McCrum, *My Year Off,* 173.
31. McCrum, *My Year Off,* 173.
32. Middlebrook, *Seeing the Crab,* 66.
33. Middlebrook, *Seeing the Crab,* 70.
34. Middlebrook, *Seeing the Crab,* 70.
35. Middlebrook, *Seeing the Crab,* 72.
36. Gilda Radner, *It's Always Something* (New York: Avon, 1989), 150.
37. McCrum, *My Year Off,* 151.
38. Hull, *Touching the Rock,* 54.
39. Hull, *Touching the Rock,* 45.
40. Hull, *Touching the Rock,* 53.
41. Diamond, *Cowards Get Cancer,* viii.
42. Diamond, *Cowards Get Cancer,* 131.
43. Diamond, *Cowards Get Cancer,* 131.

44. Diamond, *Cowards Get Cancer*, 139.
45. Bauby, *Diving Bell*, 4.
46. Bauby, *Diving Bell*, 25.
47. Bauby, *Diving Bell*, 17.
48. Bauby, *Diving Bell*, 17.
49. Bauby, *Diving Bell*, 82.
50. Bauby, *Diving Bell*, 84.
51. Bauby, *Diving Bell*, 86–87.

Chapter 4

1. Sontag, *Illness as Metaphor*, 5.
2. Sontag, *Illness as Metaphor*, 65.
3. Sontag, *Illness as Metaphor*, 3.
4. Mairs, *Waist-High*, 47–48.
5. Diamond, *Cowards Get Cancer*, 52.
6. Ehrenreich, "Welcome to Cancerland," 48.
7. Ehrenreich, "Welcome to Cancerland," 48.
8. Kleege, *Sight Unseen*, 21.
9. Kleege, *Sight Unseen*, 21.
10. Mairs, *Waist-High*, 57.
11. Murphy, *The Body Silent*, 3.
12. Kriegel, "The Body of Imagination," 26.
13. Price, *A Whole New Life*, 98.
14. Diamond, *Cowards Get Cancer*, 57.
15. Middlebrook, *Seeing the Crab*, 7.
16. William Styron, *Darkness Visible: A Memoir of Madness* (New York: Vintage, 1992), 46–47.
17. Kriegel, "The Body of Imagination," 26.
18. Broyard, *Intoxicated by My Illness*, 18.
19. Lipsyte, *Country of Illness*, 84–85.
20. Sontag, *Illness as Metaphor*, 93.
21. Sontag, *Illness as Metaphor*, 102.
22. Susanna Kaysen, *The Camera My Mother Gave Me* (New York: Alfred A. Knopf, 2001).
23. Kaysen, *Camera*, 3.
24. Kaysen, *Camera*, 11.
25. Broyard, *Intoxicated by My Illness*, 21.
26. Broyard, *Intoxicated by My Illness*, 27.
27. Broyard, *Intoxicated by My Illness*, 25.
28. Broyard, *Intoxicated by My Illness*, 41.
29. Broyard, *Intoxicated by My Illness*, 42.

30. Broyard, *Intoxicated by My Illness*, 97.
31. Broyard, *Intoxicated by My Illness*, 97.
32. Daudet, *In the Land of Pain*, 15.
33. Daudet, *In the Land of Pain*, 6.
34. Daudet, *In the Land of Pain*, 21.
35. Daudet, *In the Land of Pain*, 10.
36. Daudet, *In the Land of Pain*, 41–42.
37. Daudet, *In the Land of Pain*, 45.
38. Daudet, *In the Land of Pain*, 5.
39. Daudet, *In the Land of Pain*, 14.
40. Elaine Scarry, *The Body in Pain: The Making and Unmaking of the World* (New York: Oxford University Press, 1985), 3.
41. Scarry, *The Body in Pain*, 5.
42. Woolf, quoted in Scarry, *The Body in Pain*, 4.
43. Woolf, quoted in Scarry, *The Body in Pain*, 4.
44. Scarry, *The Body in Pain*, 5.
45. Paul Monette, *Borrowed Time* (New York: Harcourt Brace Jovanovich, 1988), 259.
46. Monette, *Borrowed Time*, 259.
47. Price, *A Whole New Life*, 160.
48. Virginia Woolf, diary entry, February 11, 1928, quoted by Hermione Lee, *Virginia Woolf* (New York: Vintage, 1999), 182.
49. Woolf, quoted in Lee, *Virginia Woolf*, 183.
50. Woolf, quoted in Lee, *Virginia Woolf*, 183.
51. Woolf, quoted in Lee, *Virginia Woolf*, 183.
52. Woolf, *On Being Ill*, 7.
53. Mairs *Waist-High*, 18.
54. Mairs, *Waist-High*, 58.
55. Kriegel, *Falling into Life*.
56. Sacks, *Leg to Stand On*, 80–82.
57. Verlyn Klinkenborg, "Appreciations; Spalding Interrupted," *New York Times*, March 10, 2004.
58. Styron, *Darkness Visible*, 7.
59. Styron, *Darkness Visible*, 5.
60. Styron, *Darkness Visible*, 5.
61. Styron, *Darkness Visible*, 17.
62. Styron, *Darkness Visible*, 16.
63. Styron, *Darkness Visible*, 17.
64. Styron, *Darkness Visible*, 17.
65. William James, *The Varieties of Religious Experience*, quoted in Styron, 17.
66. Solomon, *The Noonday Demon*, 16.
67. Solomon, *The Noonday Demon*, 16.
68. Solomon, *The Noonday Demon*, 88–89.

69. Solomon, *The Noonday Demon*, 16.
70. Solomon, *The Noonday Demon*, 16.
71. Solomon, *The Noonday Demon*, 17.
72. Solomon, *The Noonday Demon*, 18.
73. Styron, *Darkness Visible*, 82.
74. Styron, *Darkness Visible*, 82.
75. Styron, *Darkness Visible*, 1.
76. Styron, *Darkness Visible*, 83.
77. Styron, *Darkness Visible*, 82.
78. Styron, *Darkness Visible*, 83.
79. Sacks, *Leg to Stand On*, 84.
80. Sacks, *Leg to Stand On*, 84.
81. Sacks, *Leg to Stand On*, 86.
82. Sacks, *Leg to Stand On*, 86.
83. The images of night or darkness and another country appear often in titles of books about illness and disability: *Darkness Visible* (William Styron), *The Night-Side* (Floyd Skloot), *This Wild Darkness* (Harold Brodkey), *In the Country of Illness* (Robert Lipsyte), *In the Land of Pain* (Alphonse Daudet), *Planet of the Blind* (Stephen Kuuisisto).
84. Sontag, *Illness as Metaphor*, 3.
85. Gerard Manley Hopkins, *A Hopkin's Reader* (New York: Image Books, 1966), 76.
86. Styron, *Darkness Visible*, 82.
87. Styron, *Darkness Visible*, 82.
88. Scarry, *The Body in Pain*, 11.
89. Michael Cunningham, *New York Times*, January 19, 2003, 22.
90. Cunningham, 22.
91. Cunningham, 22.
92. Styron, *Darkness Visible*, 82.
93. Styron, *Darkness Visible*, 82.
94. Lerner, *Wrestling with the Angel*, 12.
95. Quoted in Lerner, *Wrestling with the Angel*, 15.
96. Quoted in Lerner, *Wrestling with the Angel*, 59.
97. Quoted in Lerner, *Wrestling with the Angel*, 59.
98. Quoted in Lerner, *Wrestling with the Angel*, 59.
99. Lerner, *Wrestling with the Angel*, 61.
100. Lerner, *Wrestling with the Angel*, 65.
101. Lerner, *Wrestling with the Angel*, 74.
102. Lerner, *Wrestling with the Angel*, 74.
103. Broyard, *Intoxicated by My Illness*, 109.
104. Broyard, *Intoxicated by My Illness*, 109.
105. Lipsyte, *Country of Illness*, 226.
106. Lerner, *Wrestling with the Angel*, 194.
107. Brodkey, *This Wild Darkness*, 169.

Chapter 5

1. Kleinman, *The Illness Narratives*, 49.
2. Mee, *A Nearly Normal Life*, 182.
3. Mee, *A Nearly Normal Life*, 182.
4. Mee, *A Nearly Normal Life*, 40.
5. Mee, *A Nearly Normal Life*, 40.
6. Mee, *A Nearly Normal Life*, 40–41.
7. Mee, *A Nearly Normal Life*, 214.
8. Mee, *A Nearly Normal Life*, 125.
9. Mee, *A Nearly Normal Life*, 125.
10. Kriegel, *Falling into Life*, 3.
11. Kriegel, *Falling into Life*, xii.
12. Kriegel, *Falling into Life*, xv.
13. Frank, *The Wounded Storyteller*, 97.
14. Frank, *The Wounded Storyteller*, 99.
15. Frank, *The Wounded Storyteller*, 99.
16. Elizabeth Becker, "Museum Gives Anne Frank Her Space," *New York Times*, June 12, 2003, E1 E5, about exhibit at the United States Holocaust Memorial Museum in Washington, D.C.
17. Lawrence Langer, *Holocaust Testimonies: The Ruins of Memory* (New Haven: Yale University Press, 1991), 19.
18. Langer, *Holocaust Testimonies*, 17.
19. Tim Parks, "Tales Told by a Computer," *New York Review of Books*, October 24, 2002, 3.
20. Parks, "Tales Told by Computer," 3.
21. Skloot, *The Night-Side*, 148.
22. Skloot, *The Night-Side*, 148–49.
23. Skloot, *The Night-Side*, 154.
24. Victoria Bell, *Zeno's Paradox: A Story* (self-published, 1997), 4.
25. Bell, *Zeno's Paradox*, 4.
26. Kleege, *Sight Unseen*, 4.
27. Kleege, *Sight Unseen*, 5.
28. Hull, *Touching the Rock*, ix.
29. Hull, *Touching the Rock*, x.
30. Hull, *Touching the Rock*, 163.
31. Hull, *Touching the Rock*, 163.
32. Hull, *Touching the Rock*, 164.
33. C. S. Lewis, *A Grief Observed* (New York: HarperCollins, 1961).
34. Lewis, *A Grief Observed*, 56.
35. Lewis, *A Grief Observed*, 56.
36. Lewis, *A Grief Observed*, 57.
37. Seltzer, *Raising the Dead*, 32.
38. Seltzer, *Raising the Dead*, 55–56.

39. Julian Barnes, introduction to Daudet, *In the Land of Pain*, xiv.
40. Barnes, introduction, xiv.
41. Barnes, introduction, xiv.
42. Daudet quoted by Barnes, introduction, xi.
43. Daudet, *In the Land of Pain*, 76.
44. Nancy Mairs, "On Living Behind Bars," in *Plaintext*, 125.
45. Mairs, "On Living Behind Bars," 125.
46. Mairs, "On Living Behind Bars," 125–26.
47. See Kathy Charmaz, *Good Days, Bad Days: The Self in Chronic Illness and Time* (New Brunswick: Rutgers University Press, 1991). Charmaz offers a helpful designation of three kinds of experiences with chronic illness—as interruption, when illness is short and recovery occurs; as intrusion, when it is permanent and demands considerable attention; and as immersion, when it requires that one reconstruct life around illness.
48. Woolf, *On Being Ill*, 3.
49. Woolf, *On Being Ill*, 3.
50. Woolf, *On Being Ill*, 23–28.
51. Woolf, *On Being Ill*, 27–28.
52. Woolf, *On Being Ill*, 28.
53. Donald Hall, *Life Work* (Boston: Beacon Press, 1993).
54. Hall, *Life Work*, 67.
55. Hall, *Life Work*, 67.
56. Hall, *Life Work*, 68.
57. Hall, *Life Work*, 68.
58. Hall, *Life Work*, 70.
59. Hall, *Life Work*, 116.
60. Hall, *Life Work*, 116.
61. Hall, *Life Work*, 116.

Chapter 6

1. Styron, *Darkness Visible*, 32–33.
2. Styron, *Darkness Visible*, 33.
3. Musa Mayer, *Examining Myself* (Boston: Faber and Faber, 1993), 166.
4. Jill Ker Conway, "Points of Departure," in William Zinsser, ed., *Inventing the Truth, The Art and Craft of Memoir* (NY: Houghton Mifflin Company, 1995), 161–77.
5. Conway, "Points of Departure," 164.
6. Price, *A Whole New Life*, 179.
7. Price, *A Whole New Life*, 179–80.
8. Langer, *Holocaust Testimonies*, 161.
9. Martin Gilbert, as quoted by Langer, *Holocaust Testimonies*, 162–63.
10. Langer, *Holocaust Testimonies*, 163.

11. Gilbert as quoted by Langer, *Holocaust Testimonies*, 163.

12. Lipsyte, *Country of Illness*, 239–50.

13. Mee, *A Nearly Normal Life*, 211.

14. Mee, *A Nearly Normal Life*, 212–13.

15. Mee, *A Nearly Normal Life*, 213.

16. Mee, *A Nearly Normal Life*, 213.

17. Conway, *Ordinary Life*, 251.

18. Conway, *Ordinary Life*, 264.

19. Joyce Wadler, *My Breast: One Woman's Cancer Story* (New York: Addison-Wesley, 1992), 166.

20. Wadler, "Cancer Redux," *New York Magazine*, September 15, 1997, and September 22, 1997.

21. Wadler, "Cancer Redux," 29.

22. Wadler, "Cancer Redux," 30.

23. Wadler, "Cancer Redux," 32.

24. Wadler, "Cancer Redux," 36.

25. Wadler, "Cancer Redux," 36.

26. Hall, *Life Work*, 124.

27. Hall, *Life Work*, 123.

28. Diamond, *Cowards Get Cancer*, 193.

29. Diamond, *Cowards Get Cancer*, 198.

30. Diamond, *Cowards Get Cancer*, 202.

31. Diamond, *Cowards Get Cancer*, 215.

32. Diamond, *Cowards Get Cancer*, 216.

33. Barnes, afterword to Daudet, *In the Land of Pain*, 78.

34. Barnes, afterword, 80.

35. Barnes, afterword, 80.

36. Barnes, afterword, 81.

37. Abba Kovner's collection of poems, "Sloan Kettering," quoted by Edward Hirsch in "A Never-Ending Hospital," *New York Times Book Review*, September 22, 2002, 13.

38. Hirsch, "A Never-Ending Hospital," 13.

39. Fenton Johnson, *Geography of the Heart* (New York: Washington Square Press, 1996), 16.

40. Stanley Kuntz, quoted by Hall, *Life Work*, 68.

Conclusion

1. Edward W. Said, *On Late Style: Music and Literature Against the Grain* (New York: Pantheon, 2006), 6.

2. Said, *On Late Style*, 7.

3. Said, *On Late Style*, 13.

4. David Rieff, "Illness as More than Metaphor," *New York Times Magazine*, December 4, 2005, 54.

Afterword

Since the first publication of *Illness and the Limits of Expression* in 2007 (University of Michigan Press), the number of people telling their personal stories about a vast array of illnesses and disabilities has continued to grow. Patients, relatives, caregivers, friends, and doctors are telling their stories in books and magazines, writing essays and poetry for journals and online publications, showing their photographs in exhibits. Illness stories are increasingly the subject of blogs and graphic memoirs and are performed by actors in plays and by spoken-word artists.

At the same time more and more universities are offering humanities courses on illness narratives, and medical schools are developing narrative medicine programs, designed to help students better understand the experience of illness so they can empathize with patients and help them give voice to their experiences. The very existence of these programs reflects the universality of the desire to grapple with the realities of illness.

Nonetheless, this continued and widespread interest in illness stories does not necessarily represent a coming to terms with the difficult reality of illness and death. In fact, the triumph narrative, with its insistence on positivity and a happy ending, is alive and well, particularly in mass-market magazines and online advertisements, as well as on media, advocacy, and drug company websites that solicit stories from patients. While the authors of these stories may acknowledge the devastation of illness and treatment, they still tend to emphasize restored health and lessons learned. They focus less on those aspects of the experience that feel beyond one's control, even unbearable.

As I have argued in this book, we Americans are especially likely to tell optimistic stories about illness, characterized by a belief that we can conquer anything if we only try hard enough. We want to tell a triumph story. It's the American story, and it reflects a persistent and still widespread reluctance among Americans to face the reality of illness and death. I once met an editor who told me she was proud to have never published a cancer book. When the Affordable Care Act was first proposed there was a huge uproar over the provision that would cover the cost of a discussion between doctor and patient about the patient's wishes for end-of-life care. This seeming reluctance to deal with death is mirrored by the fact that about one-third of our health care dollars goes to end-of-life care. As a culture we deem it appropriate to go to any length to prolong life, even when death is imminent. We won't talk about death, and even when it is inevitable we refuse to accept it.

So we tell stories that downplay the devastation and difficulties of illness and treatment. When I was writing this book I kept coming upon images in advertisements and the media depicting women with cancer who looked beautiful and showed no signs of illness or the side effects of treatment. Intended to sell cosmetics and medications or to attract customers to a particular hospital, these images have an insidious effect: they leave us with the alluring notion that you can be sick without its affecting your life.

An even more unrealistic image is being offered to women with cancer today. Over the last decade the book covers and titles of a number of cancer narratives suggest this story: "I was diagnosed with cancer at a young age but still managed to be sexy, glamorous, and spunky." The cartoonist Marisa Acocella Marchetto begins her book *Cancer Vixen: A True Story* (Pantheon Books, 2006) with this question: "What happens when a shoe-crazy, lipstick-obsessed, . . . single-forever, about-to-be-married big-city girl cartoonist with a fabulous life finds a lump in her breast?" Shoes, lipstick, single in the city, fabulous life—all code words for a *Sex and the City* kind of woman. On the cover is a drawing of a young woman with blond, flowing hair, sunglasses, and stiletto heels. Like a female superhero, she stands atop a large city.

In a similar vein, Geralyn Lucas writes a memoir called *Why I Wore Lipstick to My Mastectomy* (St. Martin's Press, 2005). On the cover of the paperback edition is a toned, perfectly made-up, dark-haired beauty. It is possible to purchase the DVD of the Lifetime Original Movie and the Amazon Instant Video whose cover features a glamorous blond. More recently, Kris Carr wrote a book entitled *Crazy Sexy Cancer Tips* (skirt!, 2007). Why *sexy* in the title? Certainly there is hardly a less apt description of how a person with cancer feels.

Carr's book has spawned an industry devoted to helping patients survive their cancer in the fashion of the triumph narrative. Carr went on to publish *Crazy Sexy Cancer Survivor: More Rebellion and Fire for Your Healing Journey, Crazy Sexy Diet: Eat Your Veggies, Ignite Your Spark, and Live Like You Mean It!*, and more. Recently a friend accompanied her mother, who has advanced cancer, to one of Carr's workshops. She was appalled that the workshop turned out to be a kind of pep rally where an insistence on positive thinking displaced any discussion of the reality of dying, her mother's reality. The mantra that one can control one's health is of little use to a dying person.

Although in-your-face book covers suggest that women are not afraid to tell all, in fact these images of the glamorous survivor suggest to me that the real women suffering behind these covers are being kept hidden from view. And sometimes the cover suggests a glamorous triumph story (perhaps the publisher's marketing department sees the advantage of selling cancer as sexy) when in fact the actual story is told as much more complex. In *Why I Wore Lipstick to My Mastectomy*, Lucas captures the particular difficulty of being a twenty-seven-year-old with breast cancer, including the issue of whether she can or should have children after chemo. Similarly, Marchetto grapples with real and difficult issues in *Cancer Vixen*: people say crazy things to her, she has no health insurance, and she worries her fiancé will not want to marry her.

The face or body of the ill person has largely disappeared from the very campaigns designed to raise money for cancer and other disease research. Fifty years ago the March of Dimes Foundation and other such charities built their advertising around pictures of people on crutches. Although some organizations still showcase those with a particular disease to raise funds, many recent campaigns for breast cancer funding present attractive women and use infantilizing pink ribbons to symbolize cancer. In addition, prospective donors are courted with the promise that they can support breast cancer research by shopping; a portion of their spending goes to research. It is even possible to support breast cancer research by buying Pink Top Gun Shotshells from Federal Premium Ammunition.

Paradoxically, despite the evidence that as Americans we deny or sugarcoat the reality of illness and dying, we seem possessed of an urgent desire to face what we all know are the inevitable experiences of illness, dying, and grief. The current widespread interest in illness stories demonstrates to me how strong that desire is. In various forums, discussions about illness and dying have drawn enormous audiences. More than six million people downloaded "The Last Lecture" given by Randy Pausch, a forty-seven-year-old professor who was dying of pancreatic cancer. His lecture, subtitled "Really Achieving Your Childhood Dreams," appealed to a wide audience hungry to hear from someone with thoughts about facing death. Pausch was interviewed by both Diane Sawyer and Oprah Winfrey, and his book, *The Last Lecture* (Hyperion, 2008), written with his friend Jeffrey Zaslow, sold over 4.5 million copies. Leroy Sievers, a renowned journalist who during his long career worked at CBS, ABC, and NPR, had colon cancer that metastasized to his brain and lung. Sievers discussed his cancer on NPR's *Morning Edition* and took part in a three-hour special on the Discovery Channel hosted by Ted Koppel and entitled *Living with Cancer*. On the NPR website Sievers posted a blog called *My Cancer* in which he candidly engaged with his readers about serious matters related to cancer.

So it is against this background of a society that on the one hand denies death, but on the other hand longs for an honest engagement with the realities of illness and dying, that people are trying to tell their stories. When I wrote *Illness and the Limits of Expression* my intention was twofold. First, I wished to challenge the triumph narrative, a challenge that was also taken up by Barbara Ehrenreich in her 2009 book *Bright-Sided: How Positive Thinking is Undermining America*

(Metropolitan Books, 2009). Second, I wanted to explore the possibilities and limitations involved in writing a story of illness that was more complex and open-ended than the triumph narrative. I focused primarily on book-length narratives that chronicled the actual experience of pain and suffering and acknowledged the way illness alters the self and disrupts a life. I only briefly explored the possibilities other artistic forms hold for representing illness and disability.

I recently heard the poet Marie Howe read from her collection *What the Living Do* (Norton, 1998). Many of her poems deal directly and poignantly with her brother's dying of AIDS. In a wonderful poem called "The Last Time" she relates the conversation she had with her brother the last time they had dinner together. Her brother took her hands in his and said, "I'm going to die soon. I want you to know that." The poem continues, "And I said, I think I do know. / And he said, What surprises me is that you don't. / And I said, I do. And he said, What? / And I said, Know that you're going to die. / And he said, No, I mean know that you are." Howe talked about what she called "key stories," stories that cannot be told, where there is something "unsayable" about the experiences in question. She described how the poet, while using words, actually works with the silences.

This discussion led me to consider the many contemporary poets who take advantage of the possibilities of poetry to get to the deeper experience of illness and disability. In 2011 Sheila Black, Jennifer Bartlett, and Michael Northen published an anthology entitled *Beauty is a Verb: The New Poetry of Disability* (Cinco Puntos Press, 2011). In a poem called "Las Dos Fridas or Script for the Erased" Sheila Black describes, with love and a kind of wistfulness, the girl she was before surgery corrected her crooked legs. She ends the poem with a reference to the painting *The Two Fridas* by Frida Kahlo in which Kahlo depicts her two selves—before and after her accident—with the hands of the two figures clasped together. In the poem Black says that she "knew what the picture meant: *Here she is. / Look at her; Look at her and love us both.*" A posthumous collection of poems by Jason Shinder entitled *Stupid Hope* (Graywolf Press, 2009) contains poems about his mother's illness and his own. One short poem called "Company" goes like this: "I've been avoiding my illness / because I'm afraid / I will die and when I do, I'll end up alone again."

Meanwhile, since I did the research for this book, a number of writers have written full-length personal memoirs that deal frankly and movingly with the complex experience of illness and loss. In Sarah Manguso's *The Two Kinds of Decay* (Farrar, Straus and Giroux, 2008) she recounts with intelligence and clarity the overwhelming experience of life in her twenties when she had an unpredictable and cruel disease that left her paralyzed for weeks at a time and faced with endless procedures and treatments. Believing that "Narratives in which one thing follows the previous thing are usually imaginary," she writes a nonlinear narrative in straightforward prose about the medical procedures she endured and the thoughts she had about what was happening to her. Other writers recount their experience with loved ones who are ill or dying. Joan Didion writes about her daughter's death and the loss entailed in her own aging in *Blue Nights* (Knopf, 2011). In *Kayak Morning: Reflections on Love, Grief, and Small Boats* (Ecco, 2012), Roger Rosenblatt, writing about the death of his daughter, captures in poetic prose something of the catastrophic nature of grief. Rachel Hadas writes movingly about her experience with her husband, who suffered from Alzheimer's disease, in her book *Strange Relation: A Memoir of Marriage, Dementia, and Poetry* (Paul Dry Books, 2011). Hadas shares with the reader her deep exploration of the literature that sustained her during that time. In *To Love What Is: A Marriage Transformed* (Farrar, Straus and Giroux, 2008) Alix Kates Shulman writes a haunting memoir that alternates between a description of her present experience with her husband, who suffered brain injuries, and a description of their past life together. Sayantani DasGupta and Marsha Hurst, in their edited collection *Stories of Illness and Healing: Women Write Their Bodies* (Kent State University Press, 2007), include many short first-person stories of illness and caregiving.

I've also noticed the emergence of new and exciting forms for telling the story of illness. In blogs, performance art, and graphic novels writers and artists are telling their stories, sometimes as triumph narratives, other times finding new ways to narrate or embody their pain, anger, and fear. The web is alive with illness stories. Many bloggers tell triumph stories, perhaps because that is the culturally acceptable story, or at least the one people are used to. But some try to confront the more difficult aspects of the illness experience. As I have observed in this book, this group seems to consist largely of those who tell stories professionally. Dana Jennings, a writer for the *New York Times*, wrote a blog called *Prostate Cancer Journal: One Man's Story*. In a direct and down-to-earth style the blog offers keen observations about the medical world Jennings journeyed through and talks about the inadequacy of language for describing the experience, particularly the inaccuracy of words such as *fight*, *battle*, and *survivor*. With compelling directness and honesty, Leroy Sievers used both his blog and public appearances to address topics people rarely talk about: the excruciating decision about whether or not to continue treatment, the painful conversation with his family about their life after his death.

Performance art seems to hold exciting possibilities for capturing the felt experience of living with particular medical conditions. An HBO program called *Brave New Voices* includes performances by some young spoken-word artists such as Jasmine Bailey, who speaks about her life with sickle-cell anemia, which she refers to as "the burden I carry." She points out that while the poet may use the phrase *I can't breathe* as a metaphor, for her it is a reality. She describes "living on earth but feeling like it's hell." Her performance is deeply moving in its frankness and searing evocation of her inner struggle. In his performance about Tourette's Syndrome, Devin Murphy brings his audience inside the feeling of rejection he experienced as a boy with Tourette's. The words he speaks take on deeper meaning because they are matched by the bodily movements characteristic of Tourette's.

The graphic novel, or, more accurately, the graphic memoir, has taken on illness as a subject with fascinating results. Miriam Engleberg titles her graphic memoir *Cancer Made Me a Shallower Person: A Memoir in Comics* (HarperCollins, 2006). At the age of forty-three she had breast cancer that metastasized to her brain. In addition to capturing the anxiety, despair, and fear that haunts her throughout her treatment, she bravely charts her own inability to embrace suggestions that she think positively, live in the present, and be grateful for every moment. In doing so she comes across as a believable human being. Brian Fies writes a graphic memoir about his mother's cancer called *Mom's Cancer* (Abrams ComicArts, 2006). First created as a web comic, it was posted anonymously and found an audience online. In her sixties his mother was diagnosed with lung cancer that metastasized to her brain. Fies's memoir is striking in that he depicts the experience not of a glamorous patient but of an ordinary woman and her normal, less-than-perfect family dealing with cancer. He shows his mother at her chemo treatment, complete with IVs, slightly hunched over and looking worn-out. He depicts the way tension about the situation causes conflict within the family. Because telling a story in pictures demands that the reader work at making the connection between panels, the reader is quickly drawn into the experience. Also, this form allows for more than one narrative voice. When the cartoon shows the adult children in the family all talking at once about their mother's situation, the outside narrator asks, "Why isn't Mom getting any of this?" Fies also uses visual references to represent the experience. To indicate how devastating chemo is for his mother, he uses a black background on which he draws in white disembodied body parts that look like the aftermath of a slaughter: legs, a clenched fist, an open hand, a head lying on its side. He thus references Picasso's painting *Guernica* to illustrate the devastation of his mother's cancer treatment.

In *Stitches: A Memoir* (Norton, 2009) David Small tells his story of being a fourteen-year-old who undergoes surgery for a cyst that turned out to be cancerous, although he did not learn this until later. Because a vocal cord was removed, his voice was greatly affected. His illustrations capture the feeling of early memories in a way that words could not. Many of the images are without accompanying words. They are stark and brutal in their depiction of his angry, anguished, sad, or despairing face. These images without words also effectively represent the silences forced on him by his illness and his family's insistence on secrecy. Central to his story is his angry, unloving mother, who, he later learns, was suffering from physical illness herself. She had been born with her heart on the wrong side of her chest and had only one functioning lung. Nate Powell's *Swallow Me Whole* (Top Shelf Productions, 2008) is a graphic novel about two teenage stepsiblings whose psychological problems include OCD, schizophrenia, and hallucinations. He uses his drawings to depict the characters' inner worlds. By forgoing the standard structures of language and frame, his drawings effectively convey the feeling of chaos that is emblematic of the inner worlds and altered states of the characters.

As I have demonstrated in this book, the stories I prefer are those that manage to break out of the bounds of the triumph narrative. Their authors acknowledge the terrible loss of self that illness causes. They reject the easy recovery depicted in the triumph narrative and acknowledge how illness takes over, changes them irrevocably, and alters the direction of their lives. The experience of illness does not fit into the familiar linear framework of the triumph narrative; it intrudes, disrupts, and overwhelms us. My hope, with *Beyond Words: Illness and the Limits of Expression*, is that people will continue to try in old and new forms to tell the story of illness with honesty and directness and that we, as readers, listeners, and audience, continue to explore the possibilities of written and artistic expression for representing the universal experience of illness and dying.

– Index –

acute illness, 24, 120, 132
Adorno, Theodor, 133
advertisements, 18
Aeschylus, 91
AIDS, 8, 22–23, 58, 76, 79, 85, 131, 135
  Harold Brodkey and, 15, 97
Alsop, Stewart, 54
Alzheimer's disease, 8, 105
American culture, 10, 36
  denial of illness and death in, 3, 4, 18,
    19, 38
  resonance of triumph narrative with,
    4–5, 6, 8, 18–24, 28–31, 37–38, 134
amputation, 62–63
*Anatomy of an Illness as Perceived by the
  Patient* (Cousins), 5
And the Band Played On (Shilts), 58
anger, 8, 19, 29, 46, 104
antibiotics, 12
Armstrong, Lance, 7–8
Auschwitz, 44
autobiography, theories of, 58–59
Autobiography of a Face (Grealy), 46, 51

Bach, Johann Sebastian, 94
Balance Within, The (Sternberg), 6
Barnes, Julian, 11, 111–12, 129–30
battle metaphor, 76–77, 136
Bauby, Jean-Dominique, 58, 71–73
beautiful sufferer, myth of the, 21,
  23–24
Because Cowards Get Cancer Too (Dia-
  mond), 58, 70–71, 77, 78, 127–28
Becker, Elizabeth, 105
Beethoven, Ludwig van, 94, 133–34
Bell, Victoria, 107

Bergman, Ingmar, 93–94
Bible, 90–91, 95
blindness, 30, 53, 68–70
  literary forms and, 107–9
  and triumph narrative, 31–34, 70, 85
  See also Hull, John; Kleege, Georgina;
    Kuusisto, Stephen
"blindness" (term), 77
body, alienation from, 46–52, 55
Body Silent, The (Murphy), 78
bone marrow transplant (*see* Middlebrook, Christina)
Borges, Jorge Luis, 106
Braille, 33, 34, 69
breast reconstruction, 63–64
Brodkey, Harold, 15, 22, 42, 54–55, 97
Broyard, Anatole, 15, 72, 79, 80–82,
  96–97
Buchner, Georg, 101–2

Camera My Mother Gave Me, The (Kaysen), 80
Camus, Albert, 91
cancer, 76, 79, 81, 107, 115, 136
  breast, 1, 7, 13, 21, 49–50, 62–64, 79,
    120, 124–26
  and damaged self, 41–42, 58, 70–71
  impending death from, 54, 96–97
  and triumph narrative, 6, 7–8
  and uncertain ending of narratives,
    124–26, 127–28, 129, 131
  See also bone marrow transplant; che-
    motherapy
Cancer Journals, The (Lorde), 62–64
Cassell, Eric, 103
chaos, 14, 92–93